MW01289118

(Jo.bFM ১৭৷৬)

Insanity's Shoes

My Running Trip
Through
Postpartum Psychosis

DEDICATION

To my precious soulmate, Wayne. Please know that I owe my regained sanity to you. You've been through the mill, but you've remained strong and patient. Thank you for sticking by my side even when I didn't trust you. With all my love and commitment for the future of our marriage. I can't wait to grow old with you and love that we have the privilege of sharing responsibility for our children for which God has entrusted us.

FORWARD

Yes I know it's traditionally spelled F-O-R-E-W-O-R-D but I spelled it this way to ask a favor of you. Pay this forward. After you read this book, please consider your wife, your sister, your friend, your coworker that is a new Mother or Mother to be? Let's raise awareness about postpartum illnesses. It can blindside the woman you love and, if not treated properly, can have devastating effects on herself or any of her family members. According to Postpartum International, Postpartum Psychosis affects 1 to 3 in 1000 Mothers. With this statistic, this could realistically be you, or the closest woman to you.

I have always wanted to write a book. Up to this point, I had never felt like I had anything to write about. Added to that, I did not believe I possessed the focus and determination to finish such a feat. Then I came to a place where I didn't have a choice. I needed to write a book—this book—about my crazy experience post-baby number two. I had great hope that writing about it would help me make sense of it, heal from it, laugh about it and give you a look inside the head of a woman that took a run through the streets of insanity after the birth of her second child.

It seems that so many women who have gone through something similar have chosen to keep the experience themselves. Perhaps they are ashamed. Perhaps they feel guilty or haven't yet labeled it for what it is. After all, we women are masters of feeling guilty for things that we have no control over. For those who have been here, please be honest about it, air it out and move on. I have found it very healing to talk about it and I feel responsible to share my story to raise awareness about postpartum psychosis (PPP).

There are several books about postpartum depression but not so many on PPP. I'm not a famous figure like Brooke Shields or Marie Osmond. I am just an average Mother inviting you to come along with me as I recount my bizarre, scary, and very real story about the events that preceded my hospitalization, my two week "vacation" in a psych ward, and the afterwards as I worked to assume my role as Mother again and to heal from the devastation of a temporary mental illness.

Before I begin, I would like to share some of the signs and symptoms that point to postpartum psychosis and/or depression as well as resources where support can be found.

STOP—You (the grandparent, father, aunt or uncle) are likely showing a lot of care, love and attention to the new baby. That is wonderful and very necessary. But, for a moment, STOP and turn your attention to that beautiful woman that just delivered that baby into the world. How is she?

LOOK—How is the new Mother's mood. Is she teary? Is she over-talkative? Is she sleeping too much? Is she not sleeping enough?

LISTEN—What is the new Mother saying? Is she expressing that she is worthless? Is she talking about strange things that are untrue? Do her statements have a spiritual slant? Is she trying to be a saviour—saving herself and her baby from evil forces?

I will not reinvent the wheel and explain why I ask these questions. Instead, if you can identify with any of them, I point you to the resources below simply because OB-GYNs do not specialize in postpartum mood disorders. You are better off and better served getting in touch with your family doctor or a counselor. Time is of the essence.

Postpartum Support International (PSI): 1-800-944.4PPD

www.postpartum.net

Postpartum blog: Postpartumprogress.com

SECTION 1: GUILTY

He was guilty. He was a child molester. He was an adulterer. He was homosexual. I needed to get away from him. I needed to run down the street. I needed to get my babies away from my evil husband before they got hurt.

Welcome to my world. It's a crazy one so hold on to your hats. You're going to accompany me on a "trip" that commences in my living room from my recliner, through my neighborhood, to Heaven, to jail, to a courtroom, to a psych ward, to Eureka Springs, back to reality and back to my living room recliner.

These are all the places that insanity took me. I have seen the other side and I am here to tell you a little about what it looks and feels like. I am not afraid to share my story with you. Perhaps it will help some other dear person shed their undeserved guilt and talk about their trip, too.

The vehicle that took me on this trip is called postpartum psychosis. The best definition I've found is on psychcentral.com. PPP is a temporary but serious illness characterized by delusional thinking. Teresa Twomey, a survivor of PPP and author of Understanding Postpartum Psychosis: A Temporary Madness, described it as "a different reality superimposed onto this reality." She says, "It's like watching a TV show and believing that it's perfectly normal for the actors to be speaking to you."

THE PERFECT STORM

Imagine painting a picture of a storm brewing. That is the best way to describe the precipitation of events that led up to my temporary insanity. First you have a "sky" darkened with sleepless nights from nursing a newborn baby. Then a "front" blows in from east of nowhere in the form of a sinus infection, high fever and earache. Then severe dehydration gets thrown into the mix. And we must not discount the heavy cloud full of stress that was on my plate. Let's see, I was whirling in a wind tunnel of responsibilities: helping my husband with our business, trying to be a perfect mom, an on-the-ball house manager, and a dedicated sister, friend and daughter. Oh, and let's not leave out those fragile hormones that bottom out after baby leaves the womb. And most damaging, the serious allergic reaction to a seemingly benign five-day dose of Zithromax (Z-Pack) prescribed for an upper respiratory and that ear infection.

The first sign of this storm was a flood of racing thoughts

that inundated my mind on a Sunday afternoon when my husband and little daughter left our infant son and me home for two hours, while they attended a church gospel meeting. Still suffering from the upper respiratory infection, I opted to stay home. As I sat there that afternoon, feeding baby Tuscan, I was amazed by the bolts of plans, "to do" lists, intentions, and ideas that started filling my head:

"It's my dad's birthday, I need to call him!"

"Wayne has GOT to get a different vehicle. Maybe he should just get that truck he's always wanted and lease it. I'll call Mike (my brother-in-law) and ask him about the leasing protocol."

"The Midwife told me I had to wait to run. I want to run now. It would be good for me."

"Ugh, I wish this earache would go away. I can't hear very well. Yikes, I hope I don't have a brain tumor. It's probably from too much cell phone radiation."

"Wow, I've got a lot of energy. Where did this come from? I'm up all hours of the night!"

If I hadn't had my arms occupied with holding and feeding my new baby, I would have been darting around doing this and that like a long-tailed cat in a room full of rockers. If only I'd had two hands free I would have jotted down all of these genius thoughts, revelations, ideas and plans on paper. I had energy, if only I had a way to carry out all my intentions.

I tried to settle down but couldn't. Because it was Sunday and I wanted to feel closer to God and had a moment to do so, I picked up my Bible and read a few verses and stopped. A verse jumped off the page that had a word in it that I, all of a sudden, understood perfectly. That word was "circumspect." I felt compelled to look it up in the dictionary. By definition it means: "careful to consider all." (Merriam-Webster). I started to dissect the word and figured that the first part must come from the same root as "circumference." My brain had a heyday and proceeded to associate "circumspect" with the word "circle." The circle image played itself out as a theme in the days ahead. You'll see!

MIDWIFE AND MORE

It was no coincidence. The Midwife of both of our children just happened to be at the gospel meeting where hubby Wayne and Talia went that afternoon. But The Midwife is more than a Midwife; she is a dear, caring friend whom I really respect. When she asked how I was doing with my infection, Wayne reported that I had had a fever and an earache still. She immediately offered to come over and see me for herself. After all, Tuscan and I were still under her postpartum care.

By the time she and her nurse got to our house, my racing thoughts were in full swing. I reported this right away. She stopped me in the kitchen and put her hand on my wrist to check my pulse. She and her nurse got to work. They immediately acted on their suspicion that I was severely dehydrated. Sure enough, I was so depleted of fluids that that it was hard for them to start an IV line. Once they got the line in, my body quickly took in, not one, but two bags of saline.

All the time the IV was pumping into my body, I was talking, talking, talking. I told them all that had been on my plate—the good and the bad stressors—that had contributed to my body being run down. They listened. They consoled. They sympathized. They understood. They nursed my depleted body as best they could.

Once I was rehydrated and they thought I had fully detoxed my brain, they encouraged me to get some rest, but while my body was weary my brain was still on overdrive. I suddenly felt enlightened, like I understood things better than even my closest relatives. I felt that I was leaving them behind. I was now on an elevated plateau of spirituality.

At the same time, I was confused about what had just happened. I felt like I had just come close to death with a rapid heartbeat and brief lapses in consciousness. The Midwife told me later I was catatonic a few times. I was scared but didn't want to admit it.

As soon as they tucked me into bed, I asked them what would they call my state of being at that time. What had I just experienced? They did not put a label on it, so I threw out the first thing that crossed my mind: nervous breakdown?! They kindly discouraged me from calling it that because the term "nervous breakdown" has negative connotations.

When they left the room, I had sudden and strong urge to pray. In that moment I was more spiritual, more enlightened than ever before. With that came a surge of thankfulness for The Midwife and nurse for coming to my rescue, for my family, for my relationship with God, for His Son, and for peace in my soul that would see me through this rough patch in the road.

I felt as if I had discovered prayer for the first time in my life. It was like a two-way phone conversation with no waiting for responses from the other end. I felt a flood of newfound energy, understanding and wisdom. It was exhilarating. I was living on a new, higher plane and could see clearly things that were veiled before.

After praying, I realized bed was no place for me. I had way too much new energy, I bounded out of bed and through the bedroom door in time to say goodbye to The Midwife. I remember walking down our front steps and seeing the beautiful face of my daughter, Talia. She beamed and shouted, "Mommy!" and jumped into my arms. Her pure and innocent countenance in that moment clearly read as, "I love you unconditionally, Mommy," remained in my mind for the weeks and months that followed. Her countenance represented truth when everything I had trusted in came tumbling down in my head and around me. Her face was what linked me to my real life. Her face was an image I held onto to ground me in healing in the days ahead.

WAYNE'S NEW WIFE

After the kids were asleep, I had the urge to tell my dear hubby exactly what was happening in my mind and heart. It was so bizarre. I had to share. I say "bizarre," but in the moment it was REAL—like a new and profound truth. Through tears, I told him he had a 'new wife' and that I'd had a new and different spiritual experience while praying earlier that evening. Also, I felt a stronger connection to Wayne. Having struggled off and on with depression, I felt I understood a little better some of what Wayne has experienced. Bless his heart. He listened, held me and most importantly held his tongue by not saying, "woman, you are crazy!"

It was approaching 11:00 p.m. Wayne was dead tired and was craving sleep, but I kept talking. I had so much to bounce off of him! I was flying high and couldn't come down. He was my best friend and soul mate. I had a strong urge to bring him with me on this trip. We could have a stronger understanding and connection than ever before.

We had time to talk, talk, talk—something day-to-day responsibilities deny us. I repeatedly tapped his shoulder to share new revelations. He was getting frustrated.

Finally, he fell asleep as I mustered enough sanity at that time to shut up for a few minutes at least for him to drop off.

WAYNE'S SIDE OF THE STORY

She was "my sunshine" as the song says. She had a way of bringing a positive spin to everything from a bad cough to impending taxes. It was as if she repelled negativity like oil and water. That's why I asked her to marry me. Besides feeling in every way that she was the right one...I knew every day would have some sunshine in it if Angie were my wife. So when we tied the knot on that September day in Jamaica 11 years ago, I felt like I was marrying my sunshine...and I was.

As time passed in our marriage, I came to rely on Angie as a gauge for balance in general. I tended to go overboard with most things whether it was work, health, whatever. My obsessive compulsive tendencies needed a rudder, a guide, a balance to tell me when I was over the line or pushing too hard. My faith in God helped me immensely; but it was reassuring to have a helpmate who grounded me and knew how to bring me back to center.

And so you can imagine how I felt on that night in June, less than one year ago, when my sunshine, my gauge, my soulmate...suddenly changed as though she, or I or someone else, had just flipped a switch.

She clasped her arms around me with a death defying grip and said, "You have a new wife." (My old wife was ok with me...I hadn't ordered a new bride!) Fear gripped my heart making me feel like my foundation was crumbling. What was happening? I decided to listen and not try to dissuade her. "I see things so much clearer now. I understand", she said, as though she'd just seen a vision from heaven. Until 2 a.m. she kept me up telling me about her fresh understanding.

THE MIDWIFE RETURNS

I lay in bed while the house slept. It was getting later. Sleep, the thing both my body and brain needed was not coming for me. I decided to not disturb Wayne and moved to the living room recliner. I had to talk to someone. I was excited. I was scared. Why couldn't I sleep? Why was my heart rate so fast? Was I dying? Did I have a rapidly progressing terminal illness?

Wayne saw the light on in the living room. He awoke and came to check my pulse. He looked at the clock and remembered The Midwife telling him to call him if I wasn't able to drop off to sleep. He called her right away. Wayne realized that dealing with a crazy woman was out of his league. I confessed that there was no way I was going to drop off when I was flying so high on thoughts and ideas and hormones and plans. He urged me to just relax in the chair and wait for The Midwife to arrive while he went back to bed.

The Midwife reappeared at our door shortly after

midnight, having driven an hour from her house. According to my text record on my cell phone, I had been anticipating her arrival out in the living room while all three angels in my house were sleeping. I sent her a misspelled message after hearing her pull up at 1:55 a.m. that fateful June 4th morning that read: "Wayne is asleep. I m n living room. I wi open dooe." (Interpretation: I am in living room. I will open door.)

As I awaited her arrival, I decided to jot down some of the racing thoughts and clear revelations that were swirling in my head. A bulleted point list was in progress. It was divided in half and I had marked "Before Glasses" and "After Glasses." The focus of that list was for The Midwife to ease my mind about whether or not what was happening to me was a bipolar episode. I planned to pin her down and ask her point blank if I was having a bipolar episode. I needed to know because the illness runs in my family and it was unlike anything that had happened before and deep down I was terrified. I was terrified to be diagnosed with an illness that is so mentally debilitating and socially misunderstood. She assured me that it was unlikely and probably due to my body being so depleted by the elements of "the storm."

JESUS RETURNS

I was no longer alone in the living room. The Midwife had, once again, come to my rescue. I began sharing my bulleted list with her, honestly inquiring about whether or not I was bipolar. Then something happened. I started to panic again and felt like I was about to die. While I was in the mindset of my life being nearly done, I had the delusion that Jesus returned. We were now in Heaven! I recall asking her to hold my hand and look into my eye. I had often read the verse that Jesus would appear "in a twinkling of an eye" and felt responsible for mentioning names of the people I wanted to be sure made it to Heaven. I felt I must utter their names in order for them to be included.

I said, with intensity, "do you feel like it is close?" She said "yes." I said, "do you feel like He (Jesus) is at the door?" She said "yes" and then she took hold of my hand. She was doing a great job of playing along with the mental theatrics that were manifesting themselves as prophetic words. Underneath it all, I think I had a fear of dying and this is how these deep feelings were coming to the surface.

The words of a hymn we sing at fellowship meetings, "hand clasped in loving hand," matched the scenario that was happening at that moment. To go along with my thoughts, my pulsing heart, a rhythmic rushing in my ears, dizziness and lightheadedness, I was convinced that we were caught up in the air to meet Him.

While there was a storm brewing in my head, it so happened there was a storm brewing outside. I heard the crack of distant thunder—a sure sign that the earth we had just left behind was burning up. I kept some parts of this delusion to myself because deep inside was the realization that perhaps I was the only one that recognized my surroundings as Heaven!

The Midwife strongly suggested that I get some sleep. She reassured me that she would sleep in our guest room, take care of Tuscan and his night feedings. Before I could rest, I had to reassure myself that Talia was okay. I opened her door and turned on her light. She awoke. Of course, she was overjoyed to have a wee morning surprise visit from Mommy. She was happy, chatty and smiling. This fed my "prophesy" that we were now in Heaven and Talia's "tears would be wiped away." It always killed me to see her upset. I wanted her to be happy. So I felt the need to tell her things that would contribute to a happy mood. I, in my altered mental state, told her that we were heading to Texas, which was not true. Because I couldn't stand to see her upset and wanted to preserve that Heavenly reality in my mind. She soon found out that the trip was cancelled and she would be without her Mommy and cared for by friends and extended family.

A SLEEPLESS NIGHT

I returned to our bedroom. I lay in bed tossing and turning with every crazy thought, picture and prophesy. I disturbed Wayne enough for him to go sleep in the living room. There I was left, alone in my bed dying to talk to someone. I somehow knew that I had to be alone while all the sane people slept, a few hours at least. I contented myself by praying and thinking of all the people I loved. Each person that popped in my head I was sure made it to Heaven, too. I couldn't wait for morning to come because I knew it would be the "dawn of the perfect day" and a "day that would never end" and there would be continual, joyful fellowship between all the people and spirits that were now together in Heaven.

More than anything, I couldn't wait to have a day with just my husband so that we could talk about everything. It was like I understood how Jesus must feel waiting to have rich fellowship with His Bride without worldly distractions coming between them.

The interesting thing about that early morning was that

there were several hymns going through my mind. Let me just tell you that I am not the best at memorization and so found it comforting, and a little surprising, how many verses came to me as I lay there. I remember smiling to myself. I was so happy! There were so many possibilities and so much hope for the future. Somehow, in the midst of that altered state of mind, I had peace. Was that something my mind created or was it given to me by God to get me through? Who knows?

THE PERFECT DAY

The sun finally rose. The perfect day had arrived. I hadn't gotten an ounce of sleep but it was unnecessary. We were in Heaven and sleep wasn't needed there! I started the day by leaving the bedroom and going to sit by the window to read my Bible. The window was cracked. There was a cool breeze and birds chirped outside. I smiled to myself again because, of course, the "perfect day," "the day that never ends" in Heaven had perfect weather. I remember reading the Bible that morning and it was a fresh experience. The words from Scripture jumped out of the page. Again I was comforted, as it seemed the words I was reading were all about me. I recall thinking, we are in Heaven, the words are all real now. We can see clearly now on the other side. This made me euphoric. I felt as if I were floating.

The angels finally woke up to join me in Heaven. I floated through breakfast, a shower and other menial preparations for the day. It was planned for Talia to go to school that day. The Midwife and Wayne agreed to take me to the emergency room in Springfield to get a doctor assess me. The fact that I had gotten no sleep the previous night and still had racing thoughts concerned them. This was not The Midwife's first rodeo, as she had witnessed postpartum illnesses in other Mothers. However the fact that I was "up" and did not exhibit the usual depressive characteristics puzzled her. We loaded the car and started driving Talia to school. The Midwife agreed to meet us at the hospital. I remember looking back at Talia in the car and seeking out her face. I needed to see that innocent truth that I had seen the night before. Sure enough, it was there. She still loved me. I was still her Mother. She was elated that day because the teachers were taking her and her daycare classmates swimming for the first time. She felt that she was in Heaven, too!

THE ER

Once little squirt was off to daycare, Wayne and I sped up to the Cox Emergency Room to meet The Midwife and to get another professional opinion on my behavior and sleeplessness. After a short wait, we were called back into a room and waited for a doctor. I remember the Cox ER working like a well-oiled machine. There was a revolving door of hospital helpers coming and going asking me questions and tapping notes into their computer system. Wayne and The Midwife later told me I was perched up on the exam table, like a kid, rapidly swinging my legs and jabbering away. Baby boy Tuscan was with us but I don't remember how he was acting amidst the chaos. He must have been an angel, fitting in and not fussing.

Finally, Dr. Williams came in. He observed me, asked questions of my hubby and Midwife and listened to what they had to say. When he heard that I had started taking Zithromax for my upper respiratory and ear infection, he immediately shared about the antibiotic's side effects. We were very impressed by him—his knowledge and bedside manner. He prescribed a muscle relaxant to encourage sleep and to slow my racing thoughts. As we were finishing up and because I was feeling especially chatty and lighthearted, I asked if he had read the quote by Thomas Edison? Taking for granted that everyone would know to what I was referring. He smirked and replied, "no." So I began spouting out the quote that I had carefully stenciled on the lobby wall at our wellness center: "The Doctor of the future will give no medicine, but will interest his patients in the care of the human frame, in diet and the cause and prevention of disease." Like I mentioned earlier, I could quote verses like never before. I was basking in my sharp memory!

It was a beautiful day. The weather was perfect. I wanted to just sit in the sun. So I parked myself on a bench outside the hospital and Wayne joined me. For some reason, we had brought our mail with us. I spotted an envelope containing the official title to our van. I looked over at Wayne and said "do you know what this means?" waving the document in the air. He said, "no." "It means we own this vehicle now. It's ours. If we have the title, we don't have to pay any loan payments." He sweetly smiled, raised his eyebrows and didn't say much to disagree with my profound discovery. This fed my belief once again that we were in Heaven and there were no longer pesky stressors like debt and financial burdens like car payments. This made me fly even higher.

We made a plan with The Midwife to grab something to eat at Mama Jean's, a local health food store with a cafe inside. She reminded us they serve hot and healthy lunches. We were game as our stomachs were growling. Plus, we needed to shop for some gluten- and dairy-free foods for Talia's newly developed food sensitivities. It was a lovely lunch with my favorite fermented drink to boot—a kombucha. We then embarked on our shopping adventure at Mama Jean's.

Because I was flying high, I threw way more things into the cart than I normally would. Instead of the Meyer's anti-bacterial hand soap that I intended to buy, I ended up with household cleaner. I bought enough alternative flours to last half a year. And somehow I convinced Wayne that we needed several kombucha drinks to stock in our fridge —and those things are a small fortune. Needless to say, we spent more than we needed to but money was of no concern to me. Now that I look back on that escapade I am amazed that my hubby was so agreeable. I think he was being "coached" by The Midwife to let me live in my dream world without barriers, or major stressors, encroaching on my state of mind.

After we finished our healthy food buying fest, it was time to fulfill my next fantasy. I had saved, researched and surfed the Net looking for the perfect diaper bag. They all seemed so cheesy, but one I had previously spotted at the Baglady Boutique, conveniently located across the street from Mama Jean's, was perfect! It was a classy, brown, faux alligator skin number by Kalencom. I was so anxious to buy it that I rushed out of Mama Jean's before Wayne had paid for our monster bill. Luckily, The Midwife was already in the parking lot and deterred me until Wayne came out with our groceries. If she hadn't been there, I would have crossed the busy road by myself without even looking both ways.

When Wayne came out of the store and approached the car, I announced that our next stop was Baglady Boutique! He didn't protest, so we crossed the road (in the van, thank goodness). He said he would stay in the car while I ran in to purchase my dream diaper bag. I made a beeline to the back of the store and snatched up the bag. I was so happy to finally have that thing in my hand that I decided to "celebrate" by getting something for Talia. I spotted a fancy dancy stamp thing that you could interchange with different designs and letters. And for the icing on the cake, I grabbed a purse organizer for my new bag. I didn't look at a single price tag. This splurge was so not typical of me!

I must have been taking a while because Wayne came in to the store just as I was checking out. He stood by, biting his tongue and silently witnessing the crazy splurge. I think the sales associate must have gotten a bit suspicious because she signaled to a co-worker to go to the front of the store and write down our license plate. Or maybe I just imagined that. Who knows?

THE DRIVE TO HEAVEN

By the time our shopping spree was checked off the day's "to do" list, Wayne was exhausted. He encouraged me to put my seat back and try to catch a wink. He knew my body was in dire need of sleep and the mental restoration that comes with it. We started our 45-minute drive back to the Branson. At one point on highway 65, Wayne swerved, almost falling asleep at the wheel. He looked at me right afterwards and said, "I just fell asleep." I just smiled to myself because that was supposed to happen. Wayne was supposed to "die" too and join me in Heaven in a "blink of an eye." I guess part of me realized I was alone in my state of mind of being in Heaven and I desperately wanted those that I love the most to join me in that perfect place. What a scary thought! Perhaps this is why some Mothers in this delusional state have made decisions that had tragic consequences for their loved ones.

Upon returning home I asked repeatedly, "where is Talia?" I wanted her with us to complete our family. Wayne kept trying to appease me and told me she was at school and that we would be picking her up at 4:00. He was still hoping I would get a dab of sleep. Things were starting to get a little out of control. The strange thing was that I still don't recall what Tuscan was doing on our way home nor after we arrived there. Did I nurse him? I don't recall.

Four o'clock finally rolled around and we set out to Talia's daycare to pick her up. That part of the day is a total blur in my mind. All I know is that we somehow ended up back home with our whole family reunited. To me, the day was still young and there were more wonderful things that needed to take place.

THE BARBECUE

It was my dream to host a backyard barbecue with all of our extended family in one happy place. There would be no rifts, divorce or long distance to separate us ever again. It was not in the plan though to exert any effort to prepare for that reunion. The event was just supposed to magically happen and would be a surprise to us all. What a happy thing!

There was work to do to get to that next heavenly destination. My brain told me that our whole family needed to walk around our neighborhood circle—back to my interpretations of the Bible word CIRCUMSPECT! I felt the need to come full circle, so to speak. For some odd reason, I insisted on walking barefoot and without my contacts or glasses. So, Wayne played along and we set out that early evening in the heat and walked several times around our circle. I think in my mind I had to withstand some pain by walking barefoot in order to arrive in Heaven with my family in tow. We kept going in the front door and out the back sliding glass door. Each time, I was waiting for the surprise of our family in the backyard. Remember, Talia and the rest of the family were in tow on this wild "journey." So, at one point, Talia looked up at me and said, "where are we going?" I said "Heaven." Then she cried and said, "but I don't want to go to Heaven, I want to go to Texas!" She had been looking forward to a trip to there. We had been planning it prior to my getting sick and the ear infection. Sadly, we had to cancel the trip to my sister's even before any of the psychosis set in, There was no way I was going to fly in an airplane with an ear infection, by myself, toting two babies.

At some point that day, Wayne realized he had more than he could handle with a crazy wife and two kiddos. He called The Midwife again and told her what was happening. Without hesitation she kicked into high gear realizing that lives could be in danger. Her first thought was to call another Mother, Donna. Donna had struggled with postpartum depression and lived within minutes of our house. She just happened to be a patient of Wayne's as well.

Later I learned that The Midwife called Donna and said, "I need you to go to Tompkins' house right now." Donna replied, "Um, I just put dinner on the grill. Why?" The Midwife said, "Just go to Tompkins right now." Donna asked, "is this an emergency?" The Midwife said, "yes." In her wisdom, The Midwife knew there needed to be another body present to help with the kids and to stand by until other help could arrive.

The other help came in the form of The Midwife's husband and daughter. They pulled up and were prepared to stay with us for a few days. They even loaded their vehicle with food to stock our fridge.

After backup arrived, I don't remember anything. The perfect day was coming to a close. I was beyond sanity at this point. I hadn't slept for two days. All I know is that I ended up in bed and had been given muscle relaxants, melatonin, a bath and a lot of TLC. I consider myself lucky to have had such wonderful care when I was in such a state.

SANITY RETURNS?

Sleep does wonders. Upon waking, I was back to my old self. I remember looking over at my sweet husband and saying, "that was weird." He looked very relieved and told me he was so happy I was feeling better. He told me we had help now and I could relax. He also assured me our babies were being taken care of. I stretched and smiled and decided life was really, really good. The Midwife had strongly encouraged Wayne to take a few days off work and unload his plate to be there for our kidlets and me. That was a huge positive—a dream come true, really. To top it off, Wayne turned to me and said, "guess who is coming to help us?" I couldn't guess. "Becky and Mike," he said. I was touched and in disbelief that my sister from Florida, and her husband, would drop everything—jobs and responsibilities of home—midweek and to come and help us. It was a confirmation of just how loving and unselfish they are.

I recall really loving my quiet time during those high-flying days and felt drawn to my Bible early that morning. I can't tell you now where I read but it was perfect for that day. After my devotional time alone, together, my hubby and I read a poem that I had recovered from a file drawer. It is titled "Slow Me Down, Lord." It remains an inspirational theme for this next, busy chapter of our lives as a family of four:

Slow me down, Lord

Ease the pounding of my heart

By the quieting of my mind.

Steady my harried pace

With a vision of the eternal reach of time.

Give me,

Amidst the confusion of my day,

The calmness of the everlasting hills.

Break the tensions of my nerves

With the soothing music of the sighing streams

That live in my memory.

Help me to know

The magical restoring power of sleep.

Teach me the art

Of taking minute vacations of slowing down to look

at a flower,

To chat with an old friend or to make a new one,

To pat a stray dog,

To watch a spider build a web,

Or to read a few lines from a good book.

Remind me each day

That the race is not always to the swift,

That there is more to life than increasing its speed.

Let me look upward

Into the branches of a towering oak

And know that it grew slowly and well.

Slow me down, Lord,

And inspire me to send my roots deep

Into the soil of life's enduring values

That I may grow toward the stars

Of my greater destiny.

The rest of the house awakened. The Midwife, her husband, and her daughter were like angels that had come to "carry" our family during a postpartum crisis. On this morning, they stirred up a delicious egg and sausage breakfast. After a little rest it was obvious I was acting more like myself. Everyone was extra happy and relieved that I had returned to sanity from a trip to the other side.

I remember The Midwife holing herself up in one of our bedrooms to research my case and to look into whether Zithromax was indeed a major player in my symptoms. She also suspected that my thyroid gland needed support. She carefully wrote a two-page list of recommended foods, supplements, and lifestyle modifications that were necessary for my recovery. She gave this to Wayne to give to whoever would be responsible for my care, if I was fortunate enough to remain at home until my hormone trip was over.

The remainder of that day, Wayne and I stayed in our little cocoon at home. Talia, on the other hand, was invited to go to Table Rock Lake with some of our friends. I recall doing her hair and sending her on her way. I was so happy that she had something fun to do while we relaxed. Our friends must have known we needed a quiet house, which doesn't happen with a chatty, busy little 4-year-old!

Everyone desperately wanted me to sleep more, but I couldn't make myself doze off. Then, The Midwife shared something she had read. She said that watching a movie can give your mind the break it needs and can have the same restorative benefits of sleep. Wayne and I were game to give it a try. We decided to watch Steel Magnolias. The weird thing was, every scene somehow was linked in my temporarily twisted mind to our being in Heaven and preparations for the wedding of Jesus to his bride. I didn't share this with Wayne. In my mind, the bride and groom were going to be him and me. He was Jesus. I was His bride. Don't ask me how we achieved that status!!

The day ended with a beautiful steak dinner prepared, with love, by The Midwife. The mood was quiet and peaceful, and the food delicious! I felt very well taken care of. Talia ended up spending the remainder of the day with our friends and was invited to accompany them out for Chinese food that night. We felt so grateful and indebted to perceptive friends that stepped in even when they weren't fully aware of what was going on.

This part is fuzzy but somehow I finally settled down to sleep for the night. I think they stuffed me full of sleepy tea and melatonin. The scene was set for some serious zzzz's. Everyone breathed easier and my overly exhausted and worried husband could get some much-needed rest, too. I remember The Midwife being concerned for his welfare at the same time. Wayne is one of those deeply compassionate people that will bend, bend, and bend more until he breaks. The Midwife, with her intuition, kept our family as intact as possible during the crisis. We owe her big!!

MY SISTER, THE SAVIOUR

The next day brought about a new set of positive things. Again, I was so happy. My health crisis was hardly a crisis during these days. I loved my life. I loved my family. And, Heaven was still happening in my mind.

The Midwife and her family were still camped out at our house. They were spoiling us with food, fresh from their farm—even fresh-churned butter! They were also helping take care of our precious babies. In her wisdom, The Midwife wanted me to be eating wholesome, non-processed foods to give my body the best chance for recovery and to reestablish balance.

It was on this day, in the late morning hours that the handoff occurred. My sister and hubby were on their way from the airport and The Midwife and her family were packing up their things to return home. It was a gorgeous day—unseasonably cool yet sunny with a breeze. I planted myself outside on the front steps and drank in the day. Talia came out to join me on the steps. She was her usual cheerful, chirpy self. She showed her love and affection that morning by plucking off one of the zinnias that her daddy had just planted. I can't remember whose idea it was—probably mine—to put that flower in my hair. I made a big effort to find a bobby pin and placed the flower strategically for her benefit. Maybe it was my attempt to have a special connection with her. That sweet little bonding session stayed in my mind for months to come.

There was more activity going on at the house that day. A special pH-altering water machine was being installed in the kitchen by my great uncle. Wayne had ordered it for our use, and to study to see if he could recommend it to his patients. It added to the chaos and excitement of the day. In my mind, this machine became a negative thing—but more on that later! While the machine was being installed, I slipped out the front door and sat on the front steps and smiled to myself because all the cars were lined up in the driveway in a single row. This was significant because of the mental picture I had in my head. The mental picture looked something like this: after three days, several cars would follow each other like a funeral procession and then our bodies would be caught up in the air and our cars would be abandoned, no longer necessary without the drivers. Perhaps this crazy image came from some of the ideas presented in the Left Behind book series. I had never read the books, but got their gist of them secondhand.

Though my memory is a little sketchy on the chronology of this day's events, one of the things that I remember is that, in my mind there was to be no more bodily pain in Heaven. Prior to this, my hubby had been struggling with a lot of dizziness and discomfort in his neck. So, the solution to this problem occurred right in front of me on Wayne's portable chiropractic adjusting table. My great uncle, a fellow chiropractor and mentor to Wayne, finished up his work installing the water machine and offered to adjust my husband's neck. I was elated that Wayne's physical ailments were being addressed.

THE GREAT ESCAPE

Everything started out hunky dory that Thursday. I proved to myself that I was a big girl and got ready for the day, dressed and combed my hair all by myself. For some odd reason, I never got around to putting in my contacts.

I managed to get my baby girl dressed and ready for school. Uncle Mike was given the task of delivering her to school that day. When I gave her hugs and kisses goodbye, little did I know that I would not be seeing her precious little face for over a week.

My sister, an RN, kicked into nurse mode and started in on what was recommended by The Midwife; keep me hydrated, regulate my blood sugar, unload my plate of stressors, get rest and eat good food. Several times early in the day, I remember my sister coming over to the recliner where I was sitting and forcing me to drink liquids—sometimes water, other times orange juice.

I was thankful for the help of my other sweet sibling. Although my sister, Paula, lived in Texas and couldn't be there in person, she was doing everything she could from a distance. She rush-shipped a box of her breast milk packed in dry ice for Tuscan along with some fresh, healthy granola. I was sane enough to be touched by this gesture.

After three days away from the office, Wayne had to return to work day. I was disappointed that our togetherness had come to an end. When he left the house that day, it marked the beginning of my suspicions of him. He was out of my sight now but not out of my deluded mind.

Most of the morning I spent parked in our living room recliner. I was so tired of being confined at home and felt even more trapped by having to be in the recliner feeding my baby boy. I began to resent my state of being, which brought on my need to escape.

Midway through that day, I looked over at my brother-in-law sitting at our dining table working on his computer. I started to become suspicious of him too. He did nothing out of character to justify the guilt I placed on him in my mind. I pegged him for spousal abuse, pedophilia and all such sins. So, I began fearing for my sister's safety, too. My mind shifted and started to race. My next thoughts were that my sister and I had to get away from these evil men that we were tied to and that could hurt our kids and us. My sister was almost halfway through her first pregnancy. We had to leave now as her unborn baby was in jeopardy.

That's when I bolted. I got out of the chair, holding Tuscan in my arms and slipped behind Mike through the back sliding glass door. I ran around the back of the house and down the side yard. My sister was right out the door behind me and started calling my name. I couldn't let her stop me, as I felt very legitimate in my actions.

She caught up with me at the end of the driveway and was holding a glass of orange juice in her hand. I stopped long enough to take a swig. Then forced her to drink some. I think I almost drowned her. My reasoning was that she and I had some running to do that morning. We had miles to go to get away from our husbands. I remember thinking that I had come to the clear realization before she had about how evil our husbands were. I felt sorry for her. She was so deceived.

Then I bolted again. I still had Tuscan in my arms. I ran

as fast as I could down the street. He started to cry as he sensed my anxiety. All of a sudden, I felt the urge to get some help from a neighbor. I turned left into the driveway of, my neighbor, Virgil's house. I ran into his garage and then into the house. Thankfully, his door was unlocked. I ran through his house yelling, "HELP!" I didn't see a soul so I had to keep running. When I exited out the front of Virgil's house, I saw that he had spotted me from his upstairs window. Little did I know, I picked the perfect house to barge into. Virgil was a volunteer fireman. He immediately sensed that it this was an emergency situation when he saw me running with a baby in my arms.

Virgil hopped into his truck and activated the emergency lights on top and followed me as I made my way to the next neighbor's house. Somewhere between Virgil's and the next house, I kicked off my flats and was again in my trademark barefoot state! I raced up the front porch steps of that neighbor's house and tried her front door. It was locked. No one was home. I panicked. I looked down on the welcome mat and found a pair of running shoes. Aha!

Just what I needed for my running trip. I slipped them on, not caring that they were a few sizes too small and that they were my neighbor's personal property!

Virgil had caught up with me in his truck. My sister and Mike had caught up with me on foot. I was cornered now by three people on the neighbor's porch, all of who were very concerned for Tuscan and me. They now knew they were dealing with more than they could handle.

Virgil gently coaxed me to sit down on the front porch swing to catch my breath. He drew my attention to baby Tuscan. He had a calm and soothing voice and came to sit down beside me. He told me how beautiful my baby was. At that point, I managed to breastfeed Tuscan in the midst of the crazy confusion and it served to calm both of us. Never mind that I had an audience! I immediately trusted Virgil and felt like I had a protectorate as I felt I had no one left on my side. Or was he on their side and had evil motives, too? My mind was in turmoil and I had nowhere to run.

Mike had called Wayne at work and filled him in on the desperate state of affairs on the home front. He dropped everything and raced home. I didn't want to see him. He was one of the men from whom I was running.

Meanwhile, Becky and Mike had rounded up more fluids and soup from home and tried to get me to eat. It took a lot of coaxing because I thought they were trying to poison me —part of a plot to kill me. I didn't trust anything that had come from our house, especially the water. I thought that the new water machine that was installed was part of an evil scheme that would ultimately kill me. My thinking was back to being very delusional.

Wayne arrived 20 minutes later and joined us on the porch. He tried to settle and reassure me but he wasn't the one for the job. I was past reason. He decided to call The Midwife and ask her opinion of what should be done. She urged Wayne to take me to the hospital. I asked to speak to her. She was very kind and firm and told me it was okay to go with Wayne. Thankfully, I was very agreeable to the idea of going to the hospital. I needed to get away from my life to sort myself out, I knew this much.

Everyone worked to get me loaded into a vehicle and on the way to the hospital. I looked to my sister for direction and reassurance as I was feeling very uneasy and didn't really trust anyone completely. She patiently agreed to accompany me so we both climbed into the back of our van like animals on their way to the slaughterhouse. In my mind, Wayne and Mike were conspirators and they had Becky and I where they wanted us. An image flashed into my mind of two helpless, victimized women on a long journey with no say in their final destination nor destiny with unfavorable conditions along the way—no bathroom stops, no AC, no food, no drink. Once again, the idea that we were on our way to Texas slipped back into my mind. This would, no doubt be a 10-plus hour ride in misery.

After these helpless thoughts came and went, I slipped back into a semi-sane state and we proceeded to climb into the middle seats like human beings. Side-by-side we waited for the driver of the van. That driver ended up being Wayne. No one was saying much as we started up the road toward the hospital. Later I learned that everyone was scared and uneasy about what I might do next.

Mike was in the vehicle ahead of us with baby Tuscan. We drove 45 miles in a procession to what would be my home for the next two weeks. I had no clue what lie ahead.

In my mind, it was going to be another short and sweet visit to the hospital to "check in," talk to a doctor, and return home to my life and recover there. No, 'twas not to be.

WAYNE'S SIDE OF THE STORY

At last we're past the drama, I thought optimistically that Thursday morning on my way to work. Angie's sister and husband came to be a great support the day before. Angie was glad to see them. I could tell she was still fragile, but things were on the mend. So...having my own business, I needed to get back to work. I went to work with the hope that all was better and would soon be back to normal.

At 11:15, I got a call from my brother in law. He sounded panicked. I'll never forget it.

"You need to come home right now. Angie just took off running down the road with the baby in her arms," he could hardly get it out.

"Is everyone ok?" I asked.

"Yes at this point they are; but you better get here right away."

"I'll be right there. Have you called 911?"
"They are already here."

Phew. I hopped in the van and raced towards the house. The 911 response turned out to be our neighbor. Fortunately Angie had run to his house...ran through his house, and then across the road with Tuscan in her arms the whole time barefoot. Thankfully the neighbor was a first responder. He was in his late 50's or early 60's and had a calm gentle way about him. He asked her if he could hold the baby....and she let him. When I arrived on the scene, Angie was there sitting on a neighbors porch with this man. When I arrived I could sense that she immediately viewed me as the intruder. For some reason she trusted this man and her sister much more than me. I tried not to take it personally and just kept my distance. It became very apparent that Angie needed some immediate help that none of us could give her. We needed to get her to the hospital but how? I'll never know how or why...but Angie knew she needed to go to the hospital and she didn't resist. That was the biggest blessing of that day. We drove the hour to Springfield while she asked some of the same questions over and over again with anxiety. We arrived at the ER and found her pulse rate at 130 bpm while sitting still. This appeared to be a strong reaction to the Z-Pack. Normally considered a safe antibiotic, the Z-Pack created havoc with her heart rate. As we waited for a psych consult, she wanted to make sure all the doors were open. In a very short time she was admitted to the mental health facility, shut out from the rest of the world, with no exposure to the outside.

In a way I felt like a traitor, but I knew our little family was in over its head and we had to do whatever it took to keep our heads above water. I left the hospital feeling tentative yet relieved. At least she could focus on getting well and not be overwhelmed with caring for our baby and little family.

THE E.R. NIGHTMARE

Once we arrived at the hospital, Wayne retrieved a wheelchair. Never mind that I had just run down the street! I was willing to play the game and do the hospital admission process the right way. Some young hospital techs greeted us and the bombardment of questions began. How was I feeling? How old was my baby? Did we have insurance? What kind of family history did I have? What was my recent behavior? Thankfully, Wayne was there to answer these. I was in no shape to give accurate information.

To them, I was a 33-year-old white female walk-in patient who had an apparent psych problem that began five days prior. My identity was starting to peel away. I was no longer a Mother or a sister and did not want to be a wife. I became a chart and a case for the professionals to crack.

I was instructed to give a urine specimen, change into a gown, and begin the waiting game. Wayne was still with me as we were given a room. Because I was so suspicious of him, I insisted that the door to our room be left open. I was preoccupied with the thought that he was going to kill me. In my mind, I was fighting for my life as those that loved me were fighting for my sanity.

I tried to inform the first hospital employee that would listen, as sly as I could manage, that I was in danger and they should be questioning my husband and not me! He was the one that had plans and needed to be taken into custody and away from our children and me. I recall being frustrated because my warning was not being heeded. I tried to convince them of what he was capable of—that he could hurt me. I showed them a bruise on my wrist from earlier in the week when Wayne tried to stop me from running down our front steps with baby Tuscan.

In spite of my distrust for Wayne, we killed time in the ER by talking. I should clarify that I was doing most of the talking as I was spilling out the contents of my brain full of racing thoughts and fears. Wayne listened and tried to calm me with words even though only chemicals would be the answer.

They tried to get me to eat. I was thinking that everyone

was on Wayne's team and had it out for me. They were trying to poison me. Nothing was safe to eat. They needed me to eat so that my blood sugar would be doing its job to help regulate my body, specifically my brain! I finally took a few bites but only after a lot of coaxing.

Now it was time for some body scans. They needed to take a look at my brain and my chest. I picked up on the fact that it would be a male x-ray tech taking me into the radiology room. Because I had a huge distrust and fear of men at that point, I made a special request that a female be in the room with me. They heeded my request and sent in a bored, annoyed-looking young female tech that begrudgingly fulfilled her duty to be a decoy for the situation at hand.

Once the scans were completed, it was time to go back to my room. Wayne was still there waiting for me. I was relieved he was still there although I still didn't want to be alone with him. I was growing tired and I think that Wayne and the hospital staff were breathing sighs of relief that I was finally "coming down," and ready to give my body and brain a rest. But I couldn't rest. Not with all the fearful thoughts and suspicions I had running through my head. I must have expressed this because one of the hospital staff assured me I was safe. They lowered the lights, reclined my bed and told me to close my eyes. I did, but only one of them. I had to keep one eye open to be sure my suspicions wouldn't be carried out while I succumbed to sleep.

All the while, I intermittently heard Tuscan crying. He wasn't. He had never come into the hospital. It was all in my head. I worried that his needs weren't being met. I already missed him and needed him close. I needed to nurse him and comfort him.

MY SISTER BECKY'S POINT OF VIEW

When our middle sister called to tell me that Angie was suffering from postpartum psychosis, I was in the parking lot of the gym, four months pregnant. My first thought was "What?!" No way!" I had just talked with Angie the day before and didn't detect anything unusual during our conversation—except for one topic that I would reflect on later. Angie had been her usual, positive, sunshiny self. I couldn't imagine her being mentally altered or unstable.

My second thought was the old ER nurse in me wondering why she wasn't in a hospital being evaluated and treated. However, later that evening we got more details from Wayne, and I could better appreciate the delicacy of the situation and that they had already received medical attention that day. It also made my husband and I realize that their household would need more hands on deck. With a two-month-old infant, a very active four-year-old girl, a husband that needed to work, and Angie needing to be alleviated of as many stressors as possible—the family needed help. We offered to fly up there ASAP. As we got ready to go I said to Mike, "I'm scared." "Of what?" he asked. "I've never been around Angie when she's like this." I felt very heavy and vulnerable.

We arrived at the house on a Wednesday. Angie was lying down and seemed weary but calm. She expressed appreciation that we had come, and I encouraged her to just rest while we managed the house. The Midwife filled me in on which medical and nutritional treatments had worked thus far and which hadn't—namely the antibiotic. The plan was for Angie to eat frequently to keep her glucose up. This would help her mind and body rest and heal after the combination of lack of sleep, dehydration, recent infection, and racing thoughts. She was still having a rapid pulse rate and frequently requested that I check it. The first evening went by with Mike and I getting groceries, cooking, and tending to the kids, all the while Wayne helping and keeping an eye on Angie. She slept off and on that night, better than she had previous nights.

On Thursday morning, Wayne went back to work and dropped Talia at daycare on his way. That left Mike and me at the house with Angie and the baby. I stayed in my comfortable workout clothes while doing dishes and sweeping the floor. Angie fed Tuscan and while he slept, she spent a little time in the hammock outside. When she came in, she seemed more restless and said she wanted to talk. So, I said "Sure." She said she wanted to talk to The Midwife, so I attempted to call her. I reminded Angie that The Midwife had office hours that day, which was why she didn't answer her cell phone. This left Angie feeling a little more on edge. I suggested that we go outside again and be together on the relaxing hammock. Tuscan was awake again and Angie was feeding him while sitting in the recliner. She then randomly said, "Oh I know, all of the crickets are here because Talia likes to listen to her crickets at night." At night, Talia DID listen to a noise machine that played cricket sounds; and yes some crickets had gotten into their house after a door had been left open. But Angie was trying to connect them in her mind and was my first indication of delusional thinking. Mike and I looked at each other and raised our eyebrows, but Angie and I proceeded outside with her holding Tuscan. I had my cell phone in one hand and a glass of orange juice in the other to help boost Angie's energy while we were outside relaxing.

Once we got outside, instead of going to the backyard to the hammock, Angie walked off to the side of the house. I could tell she was getting more restless and was encouraging her to go to the hammock. She said, "No. I want to run."

"Angie, why don't you have some orange juice and maybe you'll feel better. Let me carry Tuscan," I said.

She advanced further down their driveway. When I kept insisting that she stop, she finally stopped and forced ME to drink the orange juice, which I did. I could tell things were getting to a critical point. I couldn't reason with her and she wasn't able to see the danger of not handing over the baby. After I drank the juice, she proceeded to run. I ran after her—in my flip-flops, four months pregnant, on their hilly street. I called Mike and told him to come outside NOW! He went to the front door and saw me pursuing Angie and realized we were having a crisis. Mike got on the phone with Wayne and asked him to come home immediately then jumped into our rental car. I continued to pursue Angie, yelling at her to stop and let me have the baby. She veered off into a neighbor's driveway, ran into their open garage, and into the house. Seconds later she was flying out the front door. While I was in the neighbor's garage, the homeowner saw me and realized something was going on. "My sister is out of her head and just ran into your house with a baby!" I said. Angie was now sprinting off their porch and through their yard. Thankfully, this neighbor was a firefighter and swiftly took action. He jump into his truck and followed us. Angie ran into another neighbor's yard and bounded up their front steps. She sat down on a porch chair and put on some shoes that were sitting by the door. The neighbor in his truck caught up to us with his blue lights flashing. The lights and his calm, authoritative voice, finally convinced Angie to stop and responded to his request to keep sitting down and let him hold the baby. I frantically called The Midwife. I told her what had happened and asked her what she thought we should do. She agreed that this was a time for more drastic measures to help Angie. When Mike arrived, he hung out to the side, sensing that too many people could potentially make the situation worse. He just sat in a chair several feet away from. I asked Angie if we could move to a porch swing to relax for a while. Then Wayne arrived. At that point we sent Mike back to the house to get more food for Angie and to retrieve the Vistaril to help Angie relax. Wayne and The Midwife stayed on the phone trying to figure out which psychiatric hospital to take her to while I kept my arm around Angie to help her feel safe. It seemed as though she trusted me more than Wayne. With the baby safe in the neighbor's arms, I continued to embrace Angie until she ate and agreed to take the medication. Angie did not protest about going to the hospital. She and I rode in the back of the minivan and Wayne drove. Mike buckled Tuscan into his car seat in the rental and followed us to the Springfield ER. Later, Wayne and I confided in each other that we were silently praying for help like we'd never prayed for it before. Help for Angie, for the rest of us, and for this hugely uncertain situation we were in. The Midwife was to meet us there and we had a whole new angle to consider;

how to feed Tuscan in Angie's absence. We had brought along some frozen breast milk, and The Midwife said she would bring some donated breast milk with her. Wayne arranged to have Talia picked up from daycare, as we had no idea how long we would be in Springfield.

While Angie was being evaluated, I watched Tuscan. Mike went to the store to get diapers and formula. When Wayne finally emerged and told us that the doctors thought Angie might be bipolar or that it could possibly psychosis related to her being postpartum. Emotionally and physically, it was stressful and relieving at the same time. Angie was safe and no one was in danger. The running was over. She could get the inpatient psychiatric help she needed now. We could breathe more deeply, but felt a huge pit in our stomachs. It was scary and a myriad of thoughts came to mind. Wow, the baby could have been dropped! What if Angie had kept running into the woods and not stopped? So glad Talia didn't watch all this happen! Will I have this after I have MY baby? What if Angie doesn't recover? Our little band went and choked down some food in the cafeteria. I knew that I had to take care of myself for the road ahead, especially for the sake of my baby, and my sister's babies.

After Angie was admitted, we were told the rules and regulations that applied to family members, the phone numbers and times that we could call her. Visitation would be twice per week and limited in time. That's when it hit us that we weren't going to see Angie for several days. Wayne said, "Okay, we are going to relax and enjoy ourselves now while you are here for our sakes and Talia's sake." And so we drove home, ate and went to bed. I took on overnight baby feedings and it soon became apparent that we were going to have to start feeding Tuscan formula, as we didn't know how long Angie would be hospitalized. Thankfully, he tolerated it well and drank from a bottle like a little champ.

We had been encouraged by the hospital staff to call Angie during telephone visiting times. It was important to help her have touch with reality and to let her to know she was loved. So, we took turns calling her; me, Wayne and our other sister in Texas. Honestly, I dreaded the phone conversations because it was not the Angie I knew on the other end of the line. She would speak in a clipped way—

not our usual, warm sister. She often asked, "How are YOU?" She seemed disoriented and asked what she was doing in the hospital. Then abruptly she would say she needed to go. It seemed best to be neutral and light-hearted about the facts of our day on the home front and I didn't want to exacerbate any of her emotional trauma by talking about feelings. The hardest part was when she would ask about the kids. It seemed like she was relieved that someone was caring for them, but it was obvious that it was painful for her to be separated from them. I felt guilt for not fully answering her questions, yet I knew she couldn't handle too much information or emotionally charged topics.

At home, we got into a routine of caring for baby, Wayne working, taking Talia to daycare picking her up, doing household chores and calling Angie. How did we "make it" during that time? One dear older lady came and stayed with us to help with the cooking and household chores, another lady brought special deliveries of goat milk for Talia, friends brought meals. We spent afternoons at The Landing in Branson feeding the ducks and crying when flute music played over the loudspeakers. We read books to a bouncing four-year-old, we cuddled a sweet baby boy, we laid on the hammock. We took deep breaths, we prayed, we read our Bibles with a raw need. We felt so thankful and humbled when we felt God's presence extra-near to us. It was truly one of the scariest experiences I have ever dealt with. It was so close to my heart and the stakes were so high for this little family—suddenly Mommy was gone at a time she was needed so badly. The experience forced all of us to look at ourselves and be honest about what our individual needs were. The take-home lesson for me was that if we take care of ourselves and get the help that we need to do that, we help everyone around us. And we can't do it alone. It also made me more thankful for my husband, who not yet a Daddy, knew just what to do. Lastly, it made me never want to take Angie's sunshiny personality for granted. All in all, it better prepared me for the beautiful and overwhelming responsibility of Motherhood like nothing else could.

SECTION 2: COMMITTED

Instead of boring you with the chronological order of events as I did at the beginning of this book, I will now just share the big chunks of memorable events and impressions I had while I was on my solo "vacation" in the mental health unit trying to regain my sanity. My eyes are now wide open to what goes on behind those barred doors.

I share the same impression of the psych ward as one of my dear friends who also "spent time" following a postpartum episode: "I have never been more freaked out in my life," she told me. There are so many scary strangers in there, most of who are coming down from drug highs or consider it a second home and a respite from homelessness.

But, it was a necessary place for me to get evened out. As you will read in the pages to come, I raged like a caged animal at first—wild and out of control. I then turned a corner, thanks to a daily diet of anti-psychotic drugs. I was like a wounded bird whose wings had to be clipped before relearning to fly right.

I spent two weeks imprisoned in a cold, sterile, lonely, impersonal space to earn back my privilege of being a wife and Mother. Although it was the hardest two weeks of my life, I am grateful for the professionals that held my hands and guided me back to sanity.

THE MADWOMAN

I threw coffee on a fellow patient. I charged the nurse's station in the wee hours of the morning. I swiped a laptop computer off of a table and onto the floor. I was a madwoman. I was not "me." I was a different, violent woman. Was it the confinement and being kept from my babies? Was my behavior caused by a hormonal imbalance? Or because I was suffering from sleep deprivation? Was it the Zithromax doing tricks on my body? To this day, I have questions about what precipitated this uncharacteristic behavior.

All I know is that my violence afforded me a one-way ticket to the acute, one-on-one observation side of the psychiatric unit. There needed to be more drastic measures to tame this out-of-control lioness. So, into the private suite I went. I was given a shot of Haldol in the hind side. Also called "Vitamin H", Haldol is an anti-psychotic drug that works to balance the brain's chemistry during psychotic episodes. Before or after drugs were introduced, I don't know, I was doing some crazy things—later I was told that I had even tried to kiss one of the male psych techs. Ugh—how embarrassing!

I vaguely recall wanting my door closed, which was against protocol. I wanted safety. I wanted privacy. I needed sleep.

After the Haldol started to do its work, I drifted off into a long, long slumber. My body had needed some serious help to get some serious sleep. Thankfully the Haldol shot hit the reset button—it reset a brain that was "stuck" in a delusional thought pattern.

In my deep sleep, I had some pretty crazy dreams. I also recall a psych tech sitting outside the door of my room. Finally, I thought, I could get some rest. I had my own room and someone standing guard. I was assured that I was okay and encouraged to sleep. And while I slept, my husband didn't.

The beloved Hispanic psyciatrist on my case phoned Wayne at work with much awaited news on my condition. "Hello, Wayne! Thees ees Doctor Gallianis! You're wife ees going to be fine," the he stated confidently.

"Good!" my husband answered with a little reservation in my voice. "How is she now?" he asked.

"She's okay. She's sleeping a lot. We gave here a Haldol shot," reported Doctor Gallianis. He went on to tell Wayne the events of the morning before I was administered the wonder drug. He told of my throwing coffee and laptops, and of my attempt to break through the locked doors. He told Wayne that I had slept for most of two days. Sleep is a wonderful healer he came to realize.

THE MORGUE

Once I came to after the drug-induced sleep, my worries returned. I had to figure out my husband's whereabouts. Was he dead? I was afraid to ask, so investigate for myself. I started my search within the acute unit. I convinced myself I had been sleeping at the end of the hallway of a morgue because I was freezing cold and I had seen no life coming from any of the other rooms. I explored, peeking into the other rooms. Which one housed my husband's body? I found one that looked like his but it was the wrong color. The body started to stir in its bed! Aha! It was hi. Had he been badly burned? If so, how could he still be alive? I reasoned in my mind that I was being held in the hospital to keep me safe and sane until I was strong enough to bear the burden of this new development!

The psych techs monitoring the hall asked what I was looking for. They started asking me questions in hopes of figuring out what was rolling around in my head.

"Where is he?" I demanded.

"Who?" a tech patiently asked.

"My husband!" I said.

They went on to explain that he had gone home. In my mind that equated to heaven. I didn't believe them. They told me he would be coming to visit on Sunday and that confirmed it! He was indeed dead and I would be seeing him at a visitation on Sunday. It all played out in my mind. There would be a casket rolled into the unit's common area and friends and family would be come to gather around and pay their respects. What I couldn't figure out was what the real story was. How did he die? Who could I trust to tell me the truth?

That's when I began asking incessant questions about the wellbeing of my babies. I was still suspicious of my husband. Had he done something to hurt our kids? If he was still alive, and guilty of hurting them, were they being hurt as I sat helpless in the hospital? Somewhere deep inside I still felt solely responsible for their safety. That's why I was less-than-friendly when he came to see me that first Sunday.

THE FIRST VISIT

I have to confess, I don't recall much from the first visit with Wayne—my devoted husband. I was pretty drugged up. Heaped onto that, Wayne was guilty of everything under the sun.

He had driven over an hour and had come alone to ensure we wouldn't have any distractions during our visit. It had been three days since my admission and he wanted to be sure I was okay and making progress.

When I saw him, I didn't welcome him with my usual smile and warm embrace. Instead I was cold and looked at him as if he were a stranger. Because he can tell it in much more color and detail than I can, I will let Wayne tell you this part of the story.

"The first visit with Angie was loaded with anticipation. Besides missing her terribly, I hoped that I could make a connection and help to focus her again. As fate would have it, the only traffic jam in the history of Interstate 65 happened on that Sunday afternoon making me 30 minutes late for the one hour allotted visiting time. I was stressed because I knew she was expecting me. When the doors automatically closed behind me, the click of the lock impressed on me I was in a very controlled and institutionalized environment. The nurse led me back to the visiting area.

There stood my wife in sweats and glasses. She had a haunted look on her face. She hugged me when I reached out to hug her. It felt so good. And that's when she firmly stated, "okay you can go now."

My heart plummeted. I hadn't been there more than 30 seconds! "Don't you want to talk," I asked hopeful.

"Okay, what do you want to talk about?" she answered in the clipped tone.

"I just want to be with you." I replied pleadingly.

That's when she stepped away and walked over to the nurse and exclaimed in my direction, "you killed the kids and you killed yourself!" Her delusion rattled around in my brain for a few seconds before I could take in what she had actually said. The nurse tried to kindly, and calmly, reason with her, but it was no use. Truth and trust were nonexistent. I was as good as a murderer or a pedophile in her eyes. I slowly walked away—my eyes downcast and a huge lump in my throat. I had just driven an hour and a half for a one-minute interaction with the love of my life and I was heartbroken. I picked up my keys and belongings from the checkout station and walked slowly to my car to make the lonely drive home.

THE WRONG SIDE

Though I was on the acute side of the unit because of my violent behavior, I was coherent enough to not want to be there. I felt isolated and imprisoned. I wanted out, and wanted out now! I went so far as to charge the door that separated the two units. I would pound on the window glass so that someone on the other side would have mercy on me and let me out. I was in Hell and the other side was Heaven. I could see the group of happier faces through the window. They were talking and, in my mind, having fellowship together. I was, on the other hand, alone in my miserable torment of thoughts and emotions.

A line of a hymn kept screaming in my head, "the door is now shut, it's too late." That hopeless feeling of being on the wrong side will forever be emblazoned in my head. This gave me a more desperate desire to live my life so that that would never be my experience in Eternity.

The staff in charge took it upon themselves to put me out of my misery. They pasted some brown paper on the door to cover the window. It did help put that scenario out of my sight and finally out of mind. I took notice of a neon pink sign posted on the wall by the door that read "CAUTION: ELOPEMENT RISK." It was a warning to staff and patients alike that patients like me were watching the doors like hawks, ready to dive through if given a chance.

MY DIAGNOSIS

For the initial stint of my hospital stay, I had no clue why I had to stay for so long. It had slipped my mind that I had signed up to be admitted. I guess I had mistakenly thought it would be a casual overnight intervention and I would be on my happy way the next day.

I started having feelings of being trapped. Was I in jail? What had I done? Was this the mentally ill wing of a prison? Why couldn't I leave if I wanted to? My fellow patients were in for reasons very different from my own. I was so confused. What weren't they telling me? At night I would lie in bed with my racing mind. During the day I was unable to rest peacefully because I was trying to solve a very complex puzzle. I learned later that PPP cases are rare in the psych unit and that many of the techs were learning about my temporary illness right along with me. I must have bugged the psych techs and nurses so much by hammering questions at them that one, caring tech finally felt compelled to shed some light on my situation.

I will never forget Tiffany. She was a kind-hearted college-age tech who had done some research in college on postpartum illnesses and their psychological trademarks. She showed up at my bed one morning with a stack of papers. It was an article from a blog, www.postpartumprogress.com, written by Katherine Stone.

Finally, I had something to explain my temporary residence in the hospital and validation for the bizarre way I was feeling, acting and thinking. It was spot on. I could identify with all of it! It was like a taking in a breath of fresh air. I will forever be grateful to Tiffany for going the extra mile and bringing something to me to read in "plain mama English." Here were the most relevant parts of the article and my personal connection to them:

KS: "You have more energy than you've ever had in your life. This is like nothing you've ever experienced, and you just had a baby! You feel great."

For me: I was euphoric. Sleep was a waste of time. I was in Heaven. It was an eternal day! But Heaven was different than what I had read. There were a lot of familiar aspects!

KS: "You feel like suddenly you understand EVERYTHING, like your brain is functioning on a new and different level."

For me: This hit me spiritually—words were jumping out of the Bible pages. My prayer life changed.

KS: "You keep hearing and/or seeing things that no one else does or that you know are not there. You may have what seem like voices in your head that won't stop no matter what you do."

For me: Definitely! But it wasn't constant. It was the voice of delusion, and then it would switch to the voice of reality!

KS: "You believe that you can't trust people or have become suspicious of your family and friends—people you always trusted prior to this."

For me: Oh yeah! My husband was guilty of everything!

KS: You believe you are suddenly unique and special in some way, have some greater purpose, mission, powers or have been possessed (however, you don't want to talk about it to anyone because you know, for whatever reason, they won't understand). Or you feel these same things are true of your baby.

For me: I was the Bride of Christ and there were times I thought Tuscan was baby Jesus!

KS: You cannot remember how to do things you knew how to do in the past—like how to make a batch of cookies, read a map, program your phone or find the doctor's office. You may also have trouble focusing, like reading or doing math or following a plot on TV.

For me: Again, my functioning came and went. I tried to give the impression that things were as normal as expected of me, but in my thoughts I was on a trip. Not until I ran from home, did my thoughts and actions coincide.

TO COURT

A real, live suit-and-tie attorney came to pay me a visit at the front end of my stay at the hospital. He really threw me for a loop. I seriously started to question whether I was in jail or in a hospital. I was barely coherent at the time so I don't remember a whole lot about our brief meeting. I do recall, however, his informing me that I would be going to court and he would be representing me. In my mind, this visit smelled a whole lot like a custody case. I had been tormented during all my free time at the hospital leading up to this legal meeting that I had somehow hurt my kiddos. Countless times, I would ask the nurses and techs whether they were alive and if they were healthy. Even after they assured me that they were well and being taken care of. But I wasn't convinced. I thought they were keeping the truth from me—trying to protect the last ounce of sanity that remained for a big, bad court case. That visit really had me shaking in my boots. That was when I really started to pray. Before that, I was afraid to kneel beside my bed for fear of what my roommate would say or do. But I had become desperate and no longer cared about how the act would be perceived.

A few days later, I was summoned by the hospital staff to meet my ride. Miraculously, I managed to remain calm and collected. I think I had some extra help and strength to accept whatever was to be in my case. The taxi driver greeted me with a warm smile and accompanied me in the elevator and assisted me into the passenger side of his car. I thanked him for coming to get me. He seemed pleasantly surprised and said, "my pleasure."

I remember being so happy to be out of confinement and away from the fluorescent lights of the hospital unit. I rolled down the window and breathed in the fresh air. I also stole a look at myself in the side mirror. With no mirrors in the psych unit, I hadn't seen my reflection in days. It startled me. I was pale, my eyes were sunken in and my face looked gaunt.

We pulled into the courthouse parking lot and for some reason the driver chose a designated space marked "Reserved for Custody Court." My heart lurched. It was time for me to face the music for my crimes. At the same moment Dr. Gallianis, my psychiatrist, and his two student followers pulled up.

In the courtroom, my attorney greeted me and invited me to sit next to him on the bench. I'm sure he could pick up on how nervous I was. Without delay, the judge entered —a woman. For this I was relieved. Why? Maybe because I was desperate to be understood and supported, and could sense that this was a "woman thing."

Dr. Gallianis took the stand and described the condition for which I had been admitted to the hospital. He stated that I was extremely suspicious of my husband and my diagnosis was postpartum psychosis. He requested the judge extend my hospital stay from the initial 96-hour hold for up to 21 days. This would allow me to undergo more treatment and therapy to balance my body and mind, and to ensure I would be able to return to a positive home environment.

While Dr. Gallianis was on the stand, I watched the judge. Several times, she made eye contact with me and gave me a warm smile. That meant a lot to me. There was compassion passing from her to me—I could feel it.

Our turn came to take the stand and my attorney asked if I would like to testify. Now that I knew this was not a custody case, and it was evident that I was a victim instead of a villain, I looked at the attorney and shrugged and said, "no contest?"

He nodded yes. The judge then looked right at me when we were being dismissed and said "good luck to you."

Whew! I had made it. What had started out, in my mind, as a court case for crimes I had committed against my children ended up being just hospital protocol.

Later, I received a court record that read the following, which justified my being detained at the hospital for longer than the initial 96-hour hold:

"Patient is acutely paranoid. Thinks husband is going to kill her. Thoughts are very disorganized. Unable to understand what is happening to her. Unable to make decisions and to take care of herself and her children."

Back to the hospital we drove. Upon my return, my fellow "inmates" raised their eyebrows and asked, "back so soon?" Yes, yes I was. And I needed a nap.

MY ROOMMATES

One of the anxiety-producing aspects of my hospital stay, from the very beginning, was the fact that I had to share a room. It made me nervous. So much so that I felt the need to sleep with one eye open. I had no idea what was running through the mind of the woman lying in the next bed.

First it was an elderly lady. I'll call her Mabel. Mabel had a lame foot. She ended up being very gentle and non-threatening. But, Mabel had a habit of stealing socks for her lame foot. The first night I ended up being one sock short of a pair. Turns out it wasn't the first incident. It gave a psych tech and me a good chuckle.

Next came "Jody." I was suspicious and wary of her at first. But she kept to herself for the most part. It appeared she had been admitted to "dry out" and regulate her chemistry after a bipolar episode. She did a lot of sleeping, as most patients did on the acute side.

When Jody sensed that I had faith in God, she shared

that she was a Jehovah's Witness. We also connected on the Motherhood level. She had two school-age children. As roommates, we ended up being cordial, but never chummy. We both were on a mission—to get out of the hospital! Jody got out a week before I did. I remember being envious when she began making arrangements on the phone to get a taxi from the hospital to a place where her husband could retrieve her. I sensed that things were not too peachy between Jody and her husband.

"Gina" was the next woman I shared a room with. Gina had a potty mouth, crossed eyes and was a little on the simple side. Poor soul. I admit I was the most suspicious of her. Perhaps because I could tell that Gina's trip away from reality might have been more permanent and unpleasant than most. I sensed some unfounded jealousy toward me and it left me feeling quite uneasy. The kind of uneasiness that your imagination can have a field day with. I was afraid she would strangle me in the night.

Gina loved to play board games. The nurses encouraged us to play games with her. I complied for a round of Skip-Bo, but had to bow out before the game was over. The

Ambien I was on to help me sleep had begun to overwhelm me with drowsiness. That and the fact Gina had gotten quite excited about my playing a game with her that she started to get a little too friendly and cozy. You never know what one will be handed in a wonderful place like the psych ward.

The last roommate I had was "Miss Priss." There's no better name for her. The first thing she did was complain that her hospital treatment was substandard. She had a pretty decent vocabulary, but got a few of her fancy words jumbled under the influence of her meds. Miss Priss was in the midst of a divorce and had a young son. She came to the hospital donning diamond earrings. To the best of my recollection, she ended up in the unit because of a love affair she had with prescription medications. She seemed to come from privilege and money and couldn't stand being put in a place with so many underlings! Miss Priss did a whole lot of beauty sleeping and our conversations were few.

Can you tell I like to study people? If it paid, I'd be a professional people watcher! For me, there's nothing quite as entertaining as trying to figure out where people come from what makes them tick.

Thankfully this pastime help preoccupy my mind while I was in confinement. I just didn't exactly picture having such an up close and personal exposure to so many women from varied, and colorful, walks of life.

During the final stretch of my stay, I found it in my heart to remember these women while I was praying. Were they praying for themselves? Regardless, it was put upon my heart to do so.

HYGIENE

Personal care was a challenge. Upon admission, I was given a hygiene basket with my name on it containing some sad quality toiletries. After you do your thing, you must return the basket to one of the psych techs to lock up in a closet. To brush your teeth, you have to ask for your hygiene basket. To brush your hair, you have to ask for your hygiene basket. To shave, you have to—oh wait. That's right! For obvious reason, there were no razors included in the basket.

You could easily pick out the patients that never bothered to ask for their hygiene basket. And then there was that one patient who had just been admitted. She looked as though she'd been living on the streets for a long time. Her scent was unbearable and her long hair was stringy and oily. I will never forget the scene of the psych techs trying to corral her into the shower room as she kicked and screamed.

I asked one of the techs why we weren't permitted to

keep the baskets in our rooms. Her response was, "you would not believe the kinds of things people try to do with those toiletries." Yikes! No further questions.

There were no mirrors, period. I had a comb to pull through my long hair and one rubber band with which to fasten my hair. At night, I would slip that precious rubber band onto my wrist so that I would have it the next day. I still had my dignity. And I guess I did a decent enough job with my hair because one of the young female techs asked if I would do her hair like I had done mine.

FASHION

Shapeless, blood red scrub tops and black bottoms were standard attire in the acute unit. Male and female "guests" had the privilege of wearing the same uniform. Talk about depressing. The attire was no help to someone who needed a self-esteem boost! Plus, what I was wearing contributed to my thinking I was in jail.

Once I was coherent enough to realize I could actually do something about my state of dress, I begged for a sweatshirt. The temperature in the unit was as cold as a meat locker. A pure, white sweatshirt arrived and I was most grateful!

I remember trying to crack the code of what the uniform meant. My mind was in overdrive. I was positive the red top meant me and the other "inmates" were guilty of murder. In my mind red equals blood. The black meant we were destined to gloom and doom because of the sins that got us to where we were.

So when the white sweatshirt arrived, it covered the

blood red. I was so relieved. Maybe there was hope for me after all. I started taking note of what the others were wearing. I realized that those with white sweatshirts were eventually moved to the other side of the unit—the better side. Maybe the white sweatshirt was my ticket to getting out of "jail."

A few days later, I started seeing people in street clothes. Wait a minute! Could we actually wear real clothes? I had to find out and tracked down a psych tech.

The psych tech dude willingly grabbed the keys to a "Personal Belongings" closet and told me that I was welcome to anything that I had worn to the hospital or that my family had brought in for me. So I started digging. It was slim pickings. There was a skirt, some undergarments that had my name written on the tags and a tank top.

When I pulled out my knee-length, floral skirt that I had worn into the hospital, the psych tech vetoed it right away. He said that knee-length skirts were prohibited in the unit. I guess this was a safety measure to protect women in the unit! So, I was back to where I started.

The tech could sense that I was pretty disappointed in what was available to me from my stash. He escorted me to another locked closet containing a box of donated clothing and told me to "go shopping." All the clothes were extra big and reeked of cigarette smoke. "Never mind," I said. I felt more contented with my clean, comfy scrubs.

I hadn't been coherent enough to know that I could request clothing. I made a mental note to ask for some decent threads during my next phone visit—something that represented my true identity. Speaking of phone visits...

PHONE TIME

There were two wall-mounted phones (remember those?) in the acute unit. But they were turned on only during designated times for incoming and outgoing calls. I recall being startled out of sleep when they jangled during the "on" hours. My room was right off the common area so I got to hear all the calls, all the one-sided conversations. There were heated conversations, emotional exchanges, and desperate requests for help from those on the outside from the poor souls on my side. I chose to lie there and eavesdrop. There was little else to do.

As I began to recover from my own mental crisis, I started to think outside of myself and made it my mission to be kind toward each psych patient I encountered. I could sense that some of the people in my unit came from awful situations. So many seemed unloved and likely tried to fill that void in their life with the wrong things. Maybe they were victims first, and then became villains? I never knew their stories, but I imagined a story attached to the body that was in the unit with me. It helped me to be compassionate.

Sometimes the jangle of the phone was a call for me. In the early days of my stay, my off kilter sleep rhythms had me asleep during evening phone hours, but the techs would come and wake me to let me know I had a call. They knew contact with the outside world was essential to my healing. I groggily, but gratefully received the calls. I don't know if I made any sense to the friend or family member that was on the other end. But I do know that I was grateful for the great effort they made to reach me. With lines often busy and the window that calls could be received made it difficult to get in touch. Bless them!

One evening, I got several phone calls. I was so happy to be remembered but at the same time I felt guilty. What about all those who hadn't received a call in days? I tried to downplay my excitement during the phone conversations, hoping not to stir up envy among my fellow patients. Was I ensuring my own safety? Probably. I knew that ill treatment and malicious acts could be stirred up by jealousy.

MEAT MARKET

I started my psych ward vacation on a Thursday. The following day I found myself at a special unit luncheon that occurred every Friday. I sensed celebration in the air. Maybe because some patients would be released before the weekend. I was a little out of it that day so don't remember in it crisp detail, but I do remember feeling very out of place.

Right away, I was very aware that I was a fresh slab of flesh at the meat market. Several lewd comments and slimy sneers were made by some of the outspoken males on the floor. This did not help my distrust or fear of men. I realized I would have to be on guard at all times. Anything could happen to me here and none of the people who cared about me most would ever know it. I was absolutely terrified.

Who could I trust? Was anyone watching out for my safety? What if some dude slipped into my room to take advantage of me?

Fortunately, I learned that several precautions were in place to ensure the safety of all patients in the unit. There were hall monitors, special mirrors, room checks every half-hour and extra psych techs present when there were several patients in one area. After several initial days of fear I started to breathe easier. I realized that the techs "had my back" and I rested a little easier. I didn't have to have one eye open at all times. Whew!

THE LAB RAT

The Haldol shot I was given shortly after my arrival was the first of many meds that would be thrown at me. I felt like a lab rat. The combinations changed several times during my two-week stay. I soon physically felt the effects of imbalanced meds. Too much of one would throw my body into a tizzy. Another would cause a side effect that would have to be counteracted with another medication. It was dizzying and disconcerting.

At the beginning of my stay I fought the barrage of pills, literally. I threw water at the poor, unsuspecting nurse who dispensed the meds for the floor. I know this behavior stemmed from my resistance to any kind of prescription pill!

These are the medications I was temporarily put on to balance my brain chemistry. I have included layman descriptions in "Plain Mama English," as Katherine Stone of postpartumprogress.com puts it:

Amoxicillin: To fight the infection that I had before

hospitalization for which I had previously taken the Z-Pack.

Ambien: To help me sleep. Made me really drowsy and zombie-like during the day.

Zoloft: Anti-depressant. There is a warning that this drug can cause thoughts of suicide. I wasn't suicidal and didn't have thoughts of suicide at all before hospitalization but once I was admitted, I couldn't stand the thought of living without my babies. I thought my separation from them was permanent so maybe I voiced this and I then was labeled "suicidal."

Ziprasidone or Geodon: Anti-psychotic used to treat schizophrenia or bipolar. Thankfully, this was just a temporary medicine needed to balance out my brain chemistry.

Congentin: Administered to counteract the side effects of the Ziprasidone.

While these pills were scary and had side effects a page long, they were necessary to get me to a better place—a sane place.

FOUR ANGELS

The Sunday visiting hour rolled around again. The possibility had been discussed, by phone, that Wayne, my sister from Texas, and my two babies would come to the next visit. Under normal circumstances, no kids under 13 are permitted on the psych unit floor. So, someone had pulled some strings and taken pity on this poor, homesick Mommy and allowed for them to meet me in a conference room just outside the unit's double doors.

It was the most precious hour and it went lightning fast. It was the only chance I got to see my Texas sister on her visit. She and her husband had dropped everything, packed up their own kids and driven 10 hours to come to my family's aid.

Talia wanted to make up for lost time. She chattered nonstop and wanted me to hold her. There was nothing I wanted to do more. She kept telling me she loved me "so, soo, sooo much and missed me." This was music to my ears but also made my heart ache. I had had a secret hope that maybe, just maybe, I would be released that day and be able to go home with those that I loved most. This was not to be.

Baby boy Tuscan was looking at me with recognition in his big blue eyes. It was as if he was saying "don't I know you from somewhere?" He had filled out so much in a week's time! Even then, I doubted that he was even my baby. I thought that my family had arranged for me to hold a decoy, someone else's baby. I still was not clear in my thinking. I feared that he would not remember me. Wayne and my sister assured me that Tuscan certainly remembered. They also said that he had adjusted well to his varied caretakers. Their words put me somewhat at ease, but as any Mommy would, in the deepest part of my heart I wanted to be the one to meet his needs. But I knew I wasn't capable at that time and had to let it go.

During the last few minutes of our wonderful visit, my sister managed to distract Talia and to lead her away from the conference room so that Wayne and I could have a few minutes alone. Despite the tired look in his eyes and the weight he had lost due to stress, Wayne looked so good to me in his Sunday best. We were being closely monitored by the psych techs so didn't feel very free to show affection, but Wayne managed to show he loved and cared for me by rubbing my feet.

My angels left me with pictures of themselves that had been taken after attending Sunday morning worship meeting that morning. They had rushed to get them developed at Walgreens before they came up to the hospital. I was touched by their effort. I would look at those pictures again and again that next week. They grounded me and made me feel less alone. They also gave me motivation to work hard to get well enough to be released.

That visit, even though it was the highlight of my two weeks at the hospital, exhausted me to the core. I went straight to my room and crashed on my bed. I could not sleep so I kept looking at my new pictures. Because sleep wouldn't come I went out to the hallway to show my pictures to the psych techs. They gave the proper "oohs" and "aaahs" about my beautiful babies!

When the high from seeing my family had passed, my

mental state went south fast. I was about to experience my

last delusion.

THE MOVIE SET

My final delusion occurred the evening after my family had visited. It was a whopper!

I was Jennifer Garner playing the role of myself in my own life. Since I played the heroine in my previous delusion—one about the big Missouri earthquake and the end of the world—it was only natural that I/Jennifer be the lead in the movie about my psychotic episode. The staff was going to break it to me, any minute, that this was all just a movie production. Nothing bad had happened. Rather, I had been "found" and my acting talent had been noticed. I was now famous.

Matthew McConaughey filled the male role. One of the techs resembled him faintly. Matthew played Wayne. In my mind, everal of the techs filled the roles of friends and family.

I sang my crazy song again and am certain I was acting quite peculiar.

Because I was celebrity, there would be a party on the

set in my honor. My closest friends and family would be showing up at any moment. I kept looking toward the door and for their arrival as the techs tried to lead me back to my room.

After the delusion had gone on a while, the techs had to "talk me down" to reality. I sensed the nurses and staff were disheartened with the step backward in my healing. I heard them conferring among themselves and agreeing that having my family visit probably brought on fatigue and, in turn, triggered the delusion.

INPATIENT SHRINKING

This mama needed some serious professional help to get her mind back in working order. Dr. Reuterfors, or Dr. Roofer as I called him, was the big-gun PhD psychologist who worked with me at the hospital. Dr. Roofer was a class act. I attended many of his group psychotherapy sessions. The sessions involved rigorous mental exercises they made my brain hurt! The "ABC Model" was drilled into my head over and over. The "A" stood for our Awareness of a problem or situation, the "B" signified our Belief about it and ourselves in relationship to it, and "C" stood for the Choice we make about it that comprise our feelings and behavior going forward.

After group therapy, Dr. Roofer followed up with each patient for one-on-one counseling. I was willing for all the help I could get! I figured that the more diligent I was in utilizing all the help that was available, the sooner I could get home. I surmised that the unit viewed those who "worked the program" more favorably.

After my stay, I was given notes from these sessions and some of the things that were reported about me.

Patient's effect was bright.

She was an active group participant.

Patient did not express suicidal ideation.

One of the gifts Dr. Roofer gave to my family was a therapy session for Wayne and me. The point was to plan for our future, get on the same page and to openly discuss foreseeable challenges to my healing. During our joint session, Dr. Roofer strongly encouraged us to:

Go to a transition place, like a weekend at a resort, immediately following my release from the hospital to spend time together before real life hit us head on.

Limit time on Facebook because Dr. Roofer felt that it brought about unhealthy stimulation or a false need to gain approval from my friends on how we live our life.

Get regular exercise.

Implement structure and a schedule.

Get adequate sleep and hire a live-in nanny for nighttime feedings.

Follow-up psychiatric and psychological treatment after discharge.

RECREATION AND DIVERSIONS

Psychiatric hospitals employ trained professionals whose sole role is to try and distract mental patients so they don't go crazier than they already are! These Recreational Therapists (RT) are responsible for engaging patients in fun and games while in confinement. Once I had gotten back on my feet mentally, I took advantage of the activities they offered.

Morning stretching was one of them. I love and strive to be an active person and so was anxious to move my body. I had never been so sedentary in my life! RT James was a crack up. As he led us through stretches, he had us rolling with laughter.

Art therapy sessions were encouraged, too. The medications they put me on made it challenging to see and to stay awake. So, in my compromised state, I managed to paint a big wooden letter "A" and another time successfully smeared some paint on a sun catcher.

Another break from boredom was music therapy. The

RTs would hand out headphones and a CD of our choosing. Then, they would offer complex coloring sheets. At first, I thought this was a way for the hospital staff to get a peek inside of the patients' heads. I tried my hardest to color in the lines with markers, but was later told by Talia that I didn't do so well at this! I remember the first time or two that I attended these sessions; I had to fight back the tears. The music did its magic of bringing emotions to the surface.

The first weekend of my confinement, the staff let the patients choose a couple of movies for a special treat. Some of the ones that were chosen hit a little close to home. The stash from which we had to choose seemed to reflect our current predicament. Patch Adams, The Bird Flies Over the Cuckoo Nest, Oh Brother Wherefore Art Thou? I felt like these movies were about us and we needed to watch them to make sense of our individual reality.

Every other day, my fellow patients parked themselves in the day area and watched the tube by the hour. I recall getting really annoyed and tired of the constant drone of the television. I wasn't accustomed to this constant intrusion and missed the sanctuary of my TV-free home.

One day during my stay, the RTs rounded up all the patients and gathered us in the activity room to play the Wii. They set up with the karaoke program and we all took turns singing or playing instrumentals. I don't know who was more entertained, the patients or the RTs!

The Friday Buffet was something I really loved. The RTs stirred it up and served us. They gave us a choice early in the week for the "theme" we wanted, like picnic fare, Mexican or Italian. When Friday lunch hour rolled around, the techs put on shower caps and plastic gloves and had us line up as they dished up our special meal. I remember thinking that there must be some reason to celebrate. It was a great way to boost morale in the unit and it was a temporary break from the hospital food.

SECTION 3: HOME AGAIN

Wayne picked me up on a gorgeous Friday afternoon. I cannot put into words the elation I felt leaving that sterile and cold psych unit, but I did have mixed feelings about leaving the professionals that had helped me heal. I had grown attached to many of the techs and nurses. I had managed to make a crude note with a pencil and paper with all of the names of the special ones. I wanted to thank them for their superior care and help during my two-week stay. I sensed that it was against protocol to give hugs, but the motherly-types ignored the rules and gave me goodbye squeezes.

THE TRANSITION

Wayne had been juggling a zillion balls on the home front. One of them was lining up a getaway weekend, in immediately following my hospital stay, in Eureka Springs, Arkansas—one of our favorite spots. It would just be the two of us, and part of my rehabilitation. A time, Dr. Roofer suggested, to reconnect after my time "away" (one week in la-la land and two in the hospital), to plan my reintroduction into our household, and to RELAX! The last thing the Dr. Roofer, Wayne and I wanted was for me to become overwhelmed and relapse under the demands of being a Mother.

From the hospital, we drove an hour south to our hometown—the same trek Wayne had made nine times in two weeks. We stopped in at our local pharmacy and walked out with over $200 in anti-psychotic prescriptions. We made a stop at home to pack a suitcase, treat myself to a good bath and reunite with my razor!

Baby Tuscan was spending the night with our

neighbors/adopted grandparents, Chris and Lynn. Wanting to see Tuscan—to kiss him, to hold him and too smell him—we paid a quick visit before we started out on our weekend retreat. It was heavenly!

On the road, I took the opportunity to bask in my relief of being out of the psych ward and back with my wonderful husband. I felt safe, loved and thankful and I had peace knowing that both of our kidlets were in safe, loving hands. All the way to Eureka Springs, Wayne and I held hands and stole glances at each other. It was hard to comprehend that we were back together—just the two of us.

When we arrived at the cabin, I was pretty tuckered out. I don't remember much of that evening, but do remember telling the family that owned and managed the cabin that I had just gotten out of the psych ward. I'm sure they didn't know what to think and I probably left them wondering what kind of character had just stumbled onto their property!

Wayne was equally exhausted. He had been stressed to the max for three weeks and his body was in a serious state of fatigue. But before rest, he carefully doled out my meds. Finally. Sweet, sweet sleep.

The next morning, we relished in the quietness on the deck of the cabin and read our Bibles together. The words were made very blurry due to the meds and had to humbly ask Wayne to read the verses for me.

By mid-morning we were ravenous. We hit our favorite Eureka Springs restaurant, Mud Street Cafe. Coffee was forbidden, so I enjoyed a two cups of decaf while we waited for our food—a healthy breakfast stack of grits, eggs, sautéed veggies, cheese and alfalfa sprouts. Yum!

With happy bellies, we strolled the hilly streets of Eureka Springs and popped into a few of our favorite, eclectic shops. But the activity that appealed to us most, was lounging by the pool. We were the only guests on property so we had the delicious pool to ourselves. We soaked in the sun and quiet, and vegged for a bit.

Then, it was time to make a strategy. Who would help us with Talia and Tuscan until a nanny was hired? Who would transport me to therapy appointments? (I was not cleared to drive while on the current dosage of anti-psychotic meds.) How would we get household chores done

—the cooking, cleaning, and laundry—while I was recovering?

After a few phone calls, some planning and a lot of desperate prayer we managed to cover the bases for the coming month. We had been offered help by a few of our loving friends and relatives. All we had to do was to ask for help and plug them into the calendar. We will forever be grateful for the way God orchestrated help for our family. We kept saying to each other on that weekend away: "we are being carried right now." It was humbling, but we were grateful.

The rest of that memorable Saturday in Eureka Springs was spent sharing quiet moments, doing a little window-shopping, eating and sleeping. Just the kind of the day the doctor ordered! Soon enough we would be faced with responsibility, work and meeting the needs of our children.

MY PRESCRIPTION FOR HEALING

The hospital psychiatrist and two psychologists, along Wayne and I formulated my prescription for healing. Is it the perfect and only mix of therapies to enable a postpartum psychosis sufferer to get back on her feet and back to everyday life? We can't say for certain, but it worked well for us and we are willing to share the simplified version here.

Daily exercise

Vitamin D (sunshine)

Quality fish oil (brain food)

Limited or no caffeine (too stimulating)

Adequate sleep

Minimal to no sugar

Water (half my body weight in ounces/day)

Writing this book

Counseling

Temporary nanny

Weekly dates with husband

Frequent connection with girlfriends

Limited Facebook time

Regular chiropractic and acupuncture

OUTPATIENT SHRINKING

My hubby searched the phone book and interviewed a few psychologists in our area. He selected Linda Coker of Community Christian Counseling for my aftercare. Linda is around my mother's age and offered me a lot of comfort after I got home. It was what I needed more than anything. I just needed to know I was okay. She offered professional expertise, but also real-life experience as a Mother. One of her biggest challenges was working with me while I was heavily medicated. During our initial session, I just about fell asleep in her armchair. She was anxious for me to get weaned off of my meds, with the help of my psychiatrist, so that she could get to know, and help, the real me! She supported me as I faced life again.

One of the first things I had to work through, and admit to myself, was that I couldn't be the one to meet all of my kids' needs. We Mothers want to wear that supermom cape. We want to be all things to all people all of the time! Linda helped me laugh off this unrealistic expectation of myself. She gave me a gift, too. She encouraged me to embrace the difficult time and relish the fact that I had a lot of help to get back on my feet. When I shared with her that I felt compelled to write about my recent and bizarre trip, she was all for it.

For over a month I anxiously waited for to meet with a highly acclaimed Branson psychiatrist. Prior to our meeting, I filled out a stack of paperwork, divulging answers to many personal questions. Inside, I was dreading the appointment. I just knew he was going to slap the ol' bipolar label on me. After all, a psychiatrist's job, so I thought, was to put each patient into a box and label the box with the appropriate mental condition and then match that condition with a medication. Thankfully my sweet and supportive husband agreed to accompany me to the appointment.

The office was quite fancy in a modern leather furniture kind of way. No wonder the initial visit was $300, I thought to myself! As we waited, I noticed a suited-up drug rep chatting up the office manager. They were planning their next lunch. It turned my stomach to witness the courtship that occurs between pharmaceutical companies and doctors' offices.

I was called in to the psychiatrist's office. Wayne and I sat side-by-side on a cushy couch while the doctor fired questions at us. He was good, thorough and professional. He told us to be patient and honest as he led us to a "label" that he had already affixed to my case. Finally, he revealed that he had surely thought I was classic bipolar because of the religious nature of my delusions, my preoccupation with thinking my husband was guilty of sexual misconduct and most importantly, my "loaded" family history. However, based on the honest answers we gave of the events leading up to my hospitalization, he couldn't complete the puzzle nor could he label me bipolar. The missing piece was that I had never had a serious depressive state—characteristic of bipolar cases. Therefore, it was agreed upon that we would keep a close eye on my progress over the coming weeks to determine if it was an isolated episode, or as my hubby and I had labeled it—"the perfect storm."

The session ended with the psychiatrist recommending

a SPECT scan for a more accurate diagnosis. A SPECT scan is a type of brain-imaging technology that measures neural activity by looking at blood flow. It can shed light on cases like Alzheimer's, depression, ADD and bi-polar. The scans are often not covered by insurance and can cost anywhere between $2,000-$4,000. The psychiatrist assured me that he could get the scan right to his desktop. My hubby and I wondered later if he got any kind of kickback on these scans and/or if he was a shareholder in the machine itself. Hmmmm.

On our drive home, Wayne and I discussed the appointment and shared mixed feelings about the SPECT scan. The scan would reveal the brain's state in just one moment in time. We agreed that the brain's landscape can change with exercise, sleep, supplements and cognitive therapy and felt that a diagnosis or label, accurate or not, could cause someone to become that thing—like a self-fulfilling prophesy. Our opinion may be controversial, and not applicable in all mental cases, but we were united in it and had peace about it.

In the psychiatrist's notes it was stated, "I do feel that the patient poses a significant risk of having future psychotic symptoms." Will bipolar be something with which I will have to contend with in the future? We will see. And though it is not easy for me to admit to the possibility of it, I must remain transparent. In the meantime, what Wayne and I CAN do is purpose to be vigilant for signs of psychotic behavior, and have the psychiatrist's phone number on speed dial!

LACTATION AND RELACTATION

If you care not to know intimate details of my story of lactation, you can skip this chapter. I feel I need to share it because it is a big part of my story.

My relationship with breastfeeding may have played a part both in my sickness and in my healing. From the first hour of Tuscan's life until the day I was admitted to the hospital, I was available to my hungry little man. I loved our bond and relished his feeding time. But, out of the chute, he made it known that he wanted me all to himself—no distractions, please! He preferred to be fed off in a quiet room, all by ourselves. I remember one evening when Tuscan was a week old and we had company over. I being my social self, entertained as a good housewife does. Little had I realized but Tuscan and "shut down!" His blood sugar plummeted, so much so, that we could hardly wake him up for a feeding. I had failed to revolve around him that evening.

Sensing something wasn't right, I texted The Midwife.

She sent her nurse, and lactation expert, to our house right away. The nurse made it clear that the situation was serious and that I had to make the decision to supplement his diet or commence with what they called a "mommy-baby sit in" where the sole mission for two to four days would be to feed, feed, feed. The sit-in would allow him to catch up. I admitted that this would be difficult, but I was willing to make the sacrifice for the health of my precious baby boy. My sweet husband bought me two special pillows for our bed so that I would at least be comfy in our seclusion.

My mom was visiting that weekend. She knows me very, very well and expressed concern for my mental health during this period. Knowing that I was a very social creature, she couldn't imagine how I would make it through mentally unscathed.

We ended up making it through and Tuscan gained weight. He impressed the nurse and Midwife with his progress. But what about me? I have asked the question more than once—did this catch-up period have anything to do with my postpartum illness? Was it then that I started to feel trapped in the Mothering role? Was I like a caged animal during the mandatory seclusion? Maybe so—who can say for sure?

DRYING UP AT THE HOSPITAL

I fed baby Tuscan faithfully until I was admitted to the hospital. My family arranged for me to have a breast pump available to me, but I was only sane enough to pump a handful of times. I could sense that the psych nurses were a little put out when I requested the machine and the privacy I needed to pump. That and the fact that I knew I had to pump and dump the drug-laced milk was discouraging. It became a defeating exercise and I gave up! I somehow had the sense that I had better take care of myself instead of worrying about feeding my absent baby. Consequently, I dried up and it made me sad. I felt like Motherhood had been stripped from me. I was no longer needed to sustain my baby. I did my best to not think about it, focusing rather on getting well and getting out

RELACTATION—MAYBE?

When I expressed my mourning over not breastfeeding anymore, several people tried to make me see the bright side. That assured me that I gave him the best I could for the first five weeks of Tuscan's life. They pointed out that he was thriving and didn't really know the difference. But I still had a hollow, sad feeling in my heart because I missed the special bond that breastfeeding fostered. I had shared that bond with Talia for nearly two years and had planned the same for Tuscan.

A few weeks post-hospitalization, it dawned on me that perhaps I could re-lactate! I was off the scary meds and the psychiatrist asked whether I planned to nurse again. He thought it might help me to heal and bond again with Tuscan. I was pleasantly surprised by his support. I had heard that re-lactating was very possible with pumping, enough good fats in the mother's diet and herbal supplements. Could this help me come full circle in my healing?

I got down to business and set out to drink Traditional Medicinals Mother's Milk tea and pump like a madwoman. Though I absolutely detest pumping, I was willing to put in the time for the benefit of my baby. I pumped faithfully, every three hours, for a week but produced very little. I was disappointed and it became a chore.

When I excitedly shared my endeavor to re-lactate with my therapist, The Midwife, and close family and friends, I was a taken aback when they were a little tight lipped. They were concerned about my mental health, as I would once again be tied down and back in the living room recliner that I had bolted from a month prior. But I was determined to prove my dedication as a Mother. I had it in my mind that breastfeeding equated to being the ultimate Mother.

Well, I got my wish. For 10 minutes one day, with the help of our nanny who is studying Midwifery, Tuscan latched and fed! I could not hold back and cried tears of joy. But, for most of the feeding, Tuscan was extremely perturbed. He looked at me like "do I have to?" He had learned that he could get a lot more, with much less effort from a bottle.

I will never forget how my therapist turned my belief about breastfeeding on its head.

"Why are you doing this to him Tuscan?" she asked?

That's when it was made clear to me that my re-lactating goal was all about me, and for me. Don't get me wrong, a Mother's milk is a superior source of nutrition for a growing baby, but in my case, a mentally healthy Mother was the greater goal. I was sliding backwards on the road to recovery by fixating on breastfeeding Tuscan again. So, I let it go and regained my freedom to continue healing.

By no means am I an expert on breastfeeding, but I want to encourage Mothers who read this to please be true to you. Do what is best in your circumstance. In all honesty, I was trying to prove something, probably to other women, that I was a good Mother. Instead, I needed to focus my efforts on regaining my balance so that I could be present and joyful in the busy and wonderful years ahead.

NANNY, NANNY (FOR MY) BOO BOO

With me on the road to recovery, there was no way Wayne would be able to juggle his patients, his business, a household, a toddler, and an infant and still remain sane himself! And so we considered hiring a nanny.

Never in my wildest dreams did I ever see our family having a nanny. Before I got sick, I had the idea that a nanny was someone who was part of a household, in a big city, and for people who had way too much money. They were full/part time parent replacements for people who held demanding jobs. But having a nanny on board ended up being crucial to my healing.

We couldn't afford to hire a nanny, but we couldn't afford not to! We looked at our expenses and cutback here and there until we came up with enough money. Wayne had set out to find help for us even before I returned home from the hospital. It was a big bill to fill. I needed full nights of sleep for my mind to continue healing and so we needed 24-hour help. The nanny would have to take the night feedings and would be required to cook, clean and care for Tuscan during the day.

For two months, Christina became a part of our household. She worked so hard for us. She cleaned, planned menus, washed piles of clothes and fed Tuscan countless bottles. I used the time she was with us to heal and to spend time away from the house exercising, writing and in therapy. I had to keep reminding myself that I needed the help. Once again, I had to swallow my pride and tell myself I couldn't do it all. To try to "do it all" before I was whole again would not earn me a medal! It was very hard to hand over responsibility for taking care of my baby and our house to hired help. I prayed for grace and help to accept it. It was encouraging to read the book of Ecclesiastes about there being a time for everything under the sun:

To every thing there is a season, and a time to every purpose under the heaven:

A time to be born, and a time to die; a time to plant, and a time to pluck up that which is planted;

A time to kill, and a time to heal; a time to break down, and a time to build up;

A time to weep, and a time to laugh; a time to mourn, and a time to dance;

A time to cast away stones, and a time to gather stones together; a time to embrace, and a time to refrain from embracing;

A time to get, and a time to lose; a time to keep, and a time to cast away;

A time to rend, and a time to sew; a time to keep silence, and a time to speak;

A time to love, and a time to hate; a time of war, and a time of peace.

A BATHTUB MELTDOWN

Let me set the scene: I was taking a bubble bath in the early days after my release from the hospital. I was alone. I felt lost. I had been stripped of my Motherhood. I was not yet capable of handling my kids by myself. I was dizzy. I couldn't see well and was having trouble getting my point across verbally. I was still on meds. I felt absolutely useless.

I had no choice but to bawl. Who was I? I certainly wasn't a Mother or a housewife. I felt like a misfit in my own household.

Wayne came into the bathroom and found me distraught. He assured me he could understand why I felt the way I did. He reminded me that I would soon be able to fill those roles again. But for now, it was time to let others help so that I could heal.

At that low point, it hit me. I can write! That is something I can do right now to help myself crawl out of that dark, confusing place. I could do it for me and for broken Mothers like me. Yes, yes! That was it.

I had a bright and hopeful lifeline that would lead me forward in a positive direction. So I threw myself into this book. It gave me a purpose when I didn't know how to fill my God-given place.

THE PRESCRIPTION MEDS

I am not a fan of pills. If there is a natural remedy that can be taken instead of a synthetic prescription pill, I am all for it. However, this experience convinced me that there is a time and place for pills. My brain chemistry was off balance and it needed a tune-up fast!

The concoction of meds I was on was tweaked several times while I was in the hospital. The winning combination finally got me stabilized enough—along with precious sleep —to leave the hospital. But, once home, and the further in my healing, it became obvious that the combination was overkill. I had all the symptoms of an overdose of the anti-psychotic and the antidepressant—blurred vision, instability, drowsiness, restless, "crawling out of my skin" feeling, irritability, facial muscle twitching, slurred speech and constipation. It was awful!

To make matters worse, I learned that my meds could not be altered until my first appointment with the psychiatrist in Branson—for which I had to wait over a month! But then I remembered the psychiatrist that prescribed my meds in the hospital saying that he was available to me by phone if I needed anything post-discharge. So, I took advantage of his being accessible and called him to let him know what I was experiencing. He coached me patiently, more than once, to taper back on some of the medications. So, by the time I met with the psychiatrist, I was off of all meds! Thank you Dr. Gallianis! I am so grateful to you for helping me be free of pills and especially, free from their terrible side effects! You inspired confidence in me even before I was released from the hospital. I remember you saying, "you are going to do great. You won't have to take these medications forever. You will be able to do all the things you love to do, just don't take on too much."

I will never forget the feeling of being wracked with side effects. They were worse in the evening and needed Wayne with me during those moments. For a week I followed the same evening routine; eat an early meal, wear out my restless muscles by taking a post-dinner walk, followed by a calming bubble bath. Then I would take my evening dose of medication and fall into bed. All that was left of the side effects was that feeling of crawling out of my skin. Wayne gently brushing my hair back from my face and some soft music treated that. I would then drift off to sleep and stay asleep until six or seven the next morning.

When the side effects were at their worst, I would be overcome with panic and think I was dying. How could I possibly have these symptoms and live a normal life? Wayne always reassured me that what I was feeling was temporary and that I would fall asleep and feel better. Sure enough, he was right. The side effects were just temporary. I did end up falling asleep, and all was bright and beautiful the next morning.

SHARING—POSTPARTUM STORIES

After writing this book I realized that I was just one woman, among many, who have a postpartum story. As it was healing and freeing to talk about my crazy trip, I wanted to give an opportunity to friends, and friends of friends, to air their postpartum stories. I was overwhelmed and helped by each one who shared. They have helped me not feel alone in this, sometimes twisting, journey of Motherhood. A journey full of interesting experiences, mostly wonderful, sometimes plain awful.

I respect these women so much! By sharing their secret stories they have proven that they are honest, brave and loved their babies through the dark experiences. Group hug!!

Supermom #1:

"I have always loved children and felt Motherhood was meant for me and would come naturally. With my firstborn, I had an easy pregnancy and delivery and the first week of his life was just great. I was tired but so full of love for this little guy and his daddy. He slept well and was laid back. Then came the second week and the beginning of a few long months. My baby turned into a very whiny and, at times, very angry baby. I was his only comfort. He wouldn't take a bottle, his thumb, a pacifier, nothing. All he wanted was me and to nurse. I began having symptoms of PPD. Every afternoon from about week two to eight; it would hit me like a truck. I'd start feeling sad and depressed. Sure, baby was a handful, but his attitude was no different in the morning or the afternoon. But for me, I just knew that every afternoon, unless I was surrounded by people, I'd begin feeling depressed. Countless times I called my best friend, bawling my eyes out. She would comfort me and tell me everything would be okay and that it was a phase and that it would pass. My parents were with me part of the time and it was easier when they were around. Dad offered for mom to stay longer to help me out, but I said I'd be fine as I didn't want to disturb anyone or admit to myself that I needed help and had some PPD issues. My husband knew I was having a difficult time. He, too, reminded me that it was a phase and that it would pass and that I was doing a great job. As with my mom and dad, I didn't want to burden him with the way I truly felt so I never really opened up to him about it. At my six-week checkup, my midwife asked if I'd experienced any PPD. Downplaying what I was feeling, I just said I'd had some baby blues and that was it. Again, I wasn't being honest with myself and was very surprised that nobody probed further. I think that most people with forms of depression downplay it at first—especially if it's not very severe. These people need to be asked the right questions and pushed a little. One of the thoughts that frequently entered my mind was, "why did we ever decide to change the way things were pre-baby? Everything was going great, we had a good marriage and a good life, why did we decide to mess with that?!" I remember wanting to shake him or hurt him to make him stop crying! It is so very difficult to write those words down and acknowledge them. I never hurt him. A few spankings at too early of an age, but that was it. I felt so helpless. You feel like you should be able to fix anything as a mom but I couldn't make him happy.

What helped me to snap out of it was being with other adults, crying in a friend's arms and being with my husband when he got off work—many days I would count down to the hour. By around week 8, the PPD magically went away. That was it, it was gone. I still had a hard time with my baby because of his crying and whining, but the depressed feelings in the afternoon stopped. With time and treatment for an undetected ear infection, Isaac himself changed. He became more mobile and happier, and he started being able to show me that he loved me. He is still a somewhat difficult child, but the terrible twos are nothing compared to the first few months. One thing that sometimes makes me feel guilty is that I never had any of those feelings with Baby #2. No PPD whatsoever. My second baby has always been happy and easy. And I have felt bad for enjoying his first few months when I didn't enjoy my firstborn's."

Supermom #2

After my second baby was born, the most difficult part for me was becoming a full-time stay at home mom. It was in late August and September when reality hit me—both kids were with me every day. I felt trapped with naps, behavior, and the effort of getting both of them out. It was so difficult to get out of the house. My social circle was gone. All my teaching friends were still teaching and everyone my age who had young kids had gone back to work. I hadn't gotten a full nights sleep in over six months, and my world was consumed by poop, eating and screaming. I experienced an indescribable loneliness. I began having hormonal issues, which I later found were related to low progesterone—setting the stage for even greater feelings of depression. I decided to join an early childhood PTA to get me out of the house and to splurge on two hours of childcare a month. Two sweet hours that I don't have a kid whining or pulling on me—two reasons I teach secondary! On other issues no one other talks about, I miscarried over the holidays. I was surprised I was pregnant (see progesterone shortage above), and while it wasn't a surprise, it was extra stress on my body and mind--however, i actually think my hormone levels are higher still than usual, so feeling a bit better.

Supermom #3

My postpartum depression started after I had Olivia, our fourth child. We had had three perfect children before that; two girls and a boy and I wanted another boy. A perfect boy. So when we were told our baby was a girl with Down syndrome my perfect world was rocked more than I could handle. Our baby had a major heart defect that required open-heart surgery at five months. I kept fairly strong until she was nine months old and then something snapped. I was lost. I couldn't concentrate and I was paranoid about everything. I was opposed to taking any kind of medication, because of my ridiculous preconceived judgment of people who took depression meds. They certainly were not for ME. I kept it all together, all the time, regardless of what was thrown at me. Well, I had a lot of growing up to do and even more to learn the hard way. After trying to medicate myself, going off and on medicines like a crazy person I ended up in a psych ward— three times. Talk about life altering. I have never been so scared and freaked out in my life. I was of course in lock down units and I tried to get out at one point, I don't remember too much—just the terrifying thoughts, hallucinations and a big dark place that I really didn't think I'd ever come out of.

Thank goodness I had an amazing, understanding husband who loves me to distraction and would do whatever it took to get me back. I had family that loves unconditionally and truly cared. I feel so bad for people going through what I have, alone. Unimaginable. So with lots of doctor visits and finding the right meds I got better. Running saved me too, I found if I ran I felt better. I found that I could run a long time at a slow and steady pace, and eventually began running half marathons! The first one I did was the best and I count it as one of the coolest things I've ever done. I wasn't prepared for the emotional part when I crossed the finish line. Maybe it was the Elton John music playing, but all I wanted to do was bawl! In that moment, it dawned on me how far I had come and I was so thankful.

Supermom #4:

I'd always dreamed of having a baby, but we were married 8 years before my dream came true. My baby boy was born in August of 2012 and I thought my life was complete and full—until three days later. It seemed like a cloud had covered the sun. I didn't really feel depressed, but something wasn't quite right. I wanted to give my baby to someone else. I felt like my life wasn't normal and I had an overwhelming feeling of needing to have my life back the way it had been. My mind was so confused. I knew, on one hand, that I didn't want to give him away, but my body was telling me I couldn't cope with the baby and everything else. That was so hard for me to accept, as I was especially fond of babies. I would ask my husband, "why do I feel this way? Why do I have to go through this, when I desperately want to love my baby and be happy?" I didn't feel free to love the baby somehow and there seemed to be something in the way. I felt so desperate! I was afraid I was going out of my mind. I worried that if that happened that I'd harm the baby or myself. We decided that something had to be done and we got a prescription for medication. Four days later I felt a lot better. But it still bothered for another six or seven months. I really had to work to control my anger toward the baby when he was crabby. To say the truth, it was a total nightmare and it seemed like I should wake up anytime and everything would be normal again. I leaned on my husband heavily. That probably helped me the most. After all, he was still the same man he was before we had our baby and the most 'normal' thing in my life. His love was still the same and steady as a rock.

INTERVIEW WITH PSYCHOLOGIST LINDA COKER

Q: In what ways does postpartum depression manifest?

A: Tears. Lots of tears. An overall feeling of sadness. I personally suffered this with my first baby. I was a nurse at the time, married to a doctor. I never dreamed it would happen to me and was totally unprepared and surprised when I couldn't stop crying after I gave birth to a beautiful, healthy baby. It's important to note that most women get postpartum depression. It is a natural response to the chemical imbalance in the body once the progesterone has left the body with delivery.

Q: How is postpartum psychosis (PPP) different?

A: Psychosis is more rare. There needs to be more awareness of PPP. These cases are mostly hospitalized. A PPP sufferer is not capable of diagnosing herself as she is out of touch with reality. The burden of truth and seeking treatment rests with the spouse or significant other. She is often easily agitated and even has hallucinations. That is why it is imperative that her treatment be inpatient immediately so that she doesn't do any harm to herself or others.

Q; What does the inpatient treatment for a PPP sufferer look like?

A: They introduce medication to set in order the chemicals in the brain that the hormones have impacted. But, the key thing is for the patient to be monitored closely because soon the body evens out and the medication is no longer needed and there can easily be an overdose of the medication.

Q: In what form does help come for postpartum illnesses?

A: Postpartum sufferers are most often referred to me by the family physician or OB-GYN. But in cases of PPP, much of the psychosis has already subsided. I often get clients that are referred to me by OB-GYNs because "mental illness" is not something they feel qualified to treat. Medication and therapy are necessary for most postpartum sufferers and often on just a temporary basis until the body chemistry is balanced. I, then, refer them to their family doctor who can prescribe a medication for depression while I counsel them. But still, there is a stigma that getting help labels the postpartum sufferer as "crazy," even if they are just seen in a counselor's office.

Q: There are silent sufferers of postpartum illnesses because many women feel that they are admitting incapability, that they would be labeled mentally ill or even put themselves at risk of losing custody of their precious children. Is this a legitimate threat for postpartum sufferers?

A: I would hope that we have come far enough that people would feel like they can ask for help. To be honest, I have seen cases when legal authorities have gotten involved and it wasn't managed well. In most cases, there has to be other red flags such as a domestic disturbance for a Mother to be concerned about legal authorities stepping into her personal life. That's why it's important to surround herself with support of family and/or be well connected in her community such as with a church group to know others and to be known. That way, there can be a loving, go-to person to take care of the children if the Mother has to be admitted. Then the children don't have to even get into "the system." I have worked with cases where I have had to be a "buffer" and work on behalf of my client when attorneys or DFS have gotten involved. In my reporting I always emphasize the positive more than the negative when presenting my client's case. It seems to help because I don't believe we can help people by repeatedly hitting them over the head with what they have done wrong.

Q; What preparation do you advise for expectant Mothers for possible postpartum symptoms after her baby is born?

A: I think it is necessary to create a postpartum plan just like a Mother creates a birth plan. It is too common and support should be put in place before an episode hits, when an expectant Mother is thinking clearly. The spouse, friends, family and fellow church members should be standing by if/when help is needed. The reality is, there is a lot of stress after the baby and that baby is going to take, take, take and give very little in return.

Q: When inpatient hospitalization is necessary for postpartum depression or psychosis sufferers, should Mothers be lumped with the rest of the psych patients, many of who may be dangerous or criminal?

A: Absolutely not. Postpartum sufferers should be treated separately. They must feel safe for their healing. Hospitals should allow the baby to be with the Mother, at least for feedings. They should at least have a private room. Also, the issues that they need to deal with, that are addressed in group therapy, are so unique compared to many of the other psych ward patients. That's why they have individual treatment plans and therefore, they should treat each case differently and create the environment within the unit that caters to healing.

Q: What loving advice do you have for a postpartum sufferer, coming from a therapist and even Mother who suffered this after your own postpartum episode?

A: It's not your fault. Don't blame yourself. I know and have heard women cast a lot of blame on themselves. It is a chemical imbalance you have no control over. It may or may not happen with your next child. The caretaker should reassure the sufferer so she doesn't feel any shame for anything she did beyond her control. Our society is tough on Mothers. There is a lot of pressure these days to breastfeed, to have a perfect house, to look sexy for your husband, to maybe work outside the home. It's just not fair to expect too much of yourself.

SICK OF STIGMAS

I hope this chapter won't sound like a rant; instead I want it to be a plea. Just because I survived postpartum psychosis and visited insanity for a bit, does not make me, or any other Mother, wear the scarlet letter "M" for "Mental" the rest of my/her life. Quite the opposite. I did not hurt my baby. I did not harm myself. I have nothing to be ashamed of. I am a good Mother and love my children deeply.

So why are there so many hurtful stigmas associated with mental illness—even those who have suffered on a merely temporary basis? By admitting that I spent time in a psych ward, hallucinated and believed some pretty strange things has seemed to create a barrier between me and some of my acquaintances, longtime friends and even family members. Either the conversation is steered in a different direction or it gets glossed over. Not everyone is comfortable with straight talk about mental illness. Maybe that well-meaning friend who just shut you down when you wanted to bring up your experience means she has teetered on the edge of insanity herself and doesn't want to revisit it or face it.

Why don't we discuss temporary experiences with mental illness like we would a struggle with diabetes or heart disease? The brain is an organ, too! It can heal with proper care and treatment, just as the pancreas or heart can.

This brings me to share with you the approach my dear grandfather took as he watched members of his family suffer with mental illness. He sought to understand the way the person thought. He devoured books on bipolar disorder and depression. He studied the way the brains of famous people like Winston Churchill worked and how they overcame obstacles to achieve great things in their lives, in spite of mental illness.

My grandfather supported and respected and loved the people in his life who had mental illness, even if he didn't completely understand them or the way they thought. I am inspired by this and wish this approach were more widely adopted. Perhaps we will get there. The more that gets admitted, talked about and even published by those of us who have been—ahem—enlightened, the better.

Now, I ask a favor of you. All of you who have, or have had, a mental illness, please air it out. For those of us that have visited insanity, even temporarily, we owe it to ourselves and to the rest of humanity to be honest and courageous, and share our experience to shed light on the workings of the brain. The more we stuff it and keep our secrets, the more mysterious and misunderstood mental illness will remain. The same goes for postpartum stories. The more we share, the less "shameful" they become.

THE BEST OF FRIENDS

I can't write this chapter without getting choked up. I have some of the dearest, most-caring friends a lady could ask for. Through their gestures, I have learned how to be a friend and to stand by when times get scary. A saying that I love seems appropriate for this chapter.

"Pity stands and stares. Compassion loves and cares."

Though my friends didn't know the whole story of what was going on, they didn't gawk and whisper. They held their tongues to preserve my dignity and got busy, in quiet ways, with what was laid on their hearts to do. Their love shown, in various ways, helped me heal and I owe them big.

Kristen

After she had tried texting me with no reply for a few days, she sensed that something was up. She and her husband live in Texas, but often come up to southern

Missouri to see relatives. Ironically, it was the same weekend after I was admitted to the hospital. She stirred up some delicious meatballs for the freezer and came to the door one afternoon. She handed them to Wayne and my sister and didn't ask one question. But, that's not all.

Later, she asked Wayne if they could do anything to help. She and her husband were willing to take an additional week of vacation to return and "stand by" to help with household needs and childcare. We were beyond touched. Humbly, Wayne and I took them up on their offer.

During Kristen's stay, she asked if I would mind if she took on the daunting task of organizing our home office. It didn't take long for me to agree to that! We had fun shopping together for coordinating file boxes, decorative labels and containers. The result was as close to a Pottery Barn catalog picture as you could get. Thank you Kristen!

Esther

Esther excels at filling in the gaps and does so quietly and without a need for recognition. She offered to drive me around when I was heavily medicated. She took me to appointments and ran errands for us. While helping us, she had a family tragedy of her own. I will never forget the tearful heart-to-heart chats we shared between a pedicure and lunch. I learned a lot from her about how to quietly stand by.

Monica

She is my favorite fitness instructor. She opened her heart and offered me what she does best—personal training. She was a real "upper" and made sure I was getting out of the house and meeting her to give my body a healthy challenge.

Audra & Elisa

These two Mommy friends are from my college days. We were roommates 12 years ago. Thankfully, we have kept in touch and remain close. When these friends caught wind of our family's predicament they called Wayne and expressed their care and concern. They sent note with a generous gift card to Whole Foods and a box with Bed Head shampoo and conditioner with which they remembered I had a love affair during our college days! A few weeks after I was discharged, the asked if they could come for a visit to support me and give hugs to our babies. Not wanting to overwhelm me, they left three of their four total babies at home with daddies and grandparents. They were true to their word and left Texas at 4:00 on a Friday morning and drove all day to spend the weekend with me. As if that wasn't enough, they surprised me with a gently used BOB jogging stroller they'd found on Craigslist! They put a bow on it and snuck it to the front door and told me that there was a delivery for me on the front step. I was ecstatic. These sweet friends know me.

Jade

Our precious, gentle, loyal employee did whatever she could. If it was diapers we needed, she came through for us. She even dropped by the house, picked me up and took me with her to yoga class when I wasn't able to drive.

Jamie

My friend Jamie has a little girl, Tyleigh, who is the same age as Talia. They are best buds. So, naturally, their mamas are pretty close, too! When I was sick, she offered to come up and kid sit. The weekend I was released and Wayne and I had our weekend alone, Talia spent the weekend with Jamie's family. Since Talia loves their family dearly, it wasn't too painful for her to be away from Daddy. On our way home from our weekend away, we surprised Talia and showed up at Jamie's house to pick her up and take her home. After the happy reunion with Talia, we were guests at Jamie's Sunday dinner table. This is a true example of what my mom always said when we were growing up "it's easy to love people who love my kids."

Susie

She came and stayed for as long as was necessary to keep things humming. She did countless dishes, took over night feedings, cooked and cleaned and made sure I was getting the rest that was prescribed.

Becki & Elliott

They invited Tuscan for a sleepover at their house! They filled in a gap and sacrificed some of their sleep to keep little guy happy!

Amber

Amber called me at the hospital nearly every evening just to check in and tell me she and her family were rooting for me. She was consistent. Not only that, she brought food to my family and took Talia under her wing before and during my hospital stay. I got a clear picture of her on the inside and saw a heart full of love and care.

LETTER TO TUSCAN

I loved you the minute I saw you. You were and are very much wanted and you complete our family. From the first time I held you, I wanted to protect you. You are a gift from God. I thank Him for you.

I had a hard time after you were born. It wasn't your fault. It wasn't my fault. My body played some funny tricks on me. I had to be in the hospital and away from you and your sweet big sister for two weeks. Being away from you both just about killed me, yet the image of your precious faces motivated me to get well and out of there. You were very lucky to have a strong Daddy, kind friends and loving family to take care of you when I couldn't.

I want to be the best kind of Mom. I want to love you the way that you deserve. I want to guide you toward the best pathway in life. I can do this, if and only if, I am being guided by God to follow the example of Jesus.

I can't wait to watch you grow. I can't wait to see you and your sister play and giggle. I can't wait to make lasting memories as a family.

Thank you for being patient with me. Thank you for your unconditional love. I am not perfect. I have and will make mistakes. I want to be patient with you, too, as you make mistakes and grow into a boy and then a man. You have an excellent example of a man in your Daddy.

With all my heart and devotion,

Your Mommy

LETTER TO TALIA

You will always be my baby girl even though you are a big sister now. Do you remember when Mommy had to be gone for two weeks when your baby brother was born? Well, I had to be in the hospital to get better. When Mommies have babies, sometimes their bodies play tricks. Some Mommy's get sad and cry. Some Mommy's say funny things that aren't true because they haven't been sleeping a lot.

I still remember you doing a puzzle quietly on the floor in front of me over and over. You are a smart girl and you were trying to figure out the pieces of the puzzle of our normal family life that wasn't quite fitting together.

The image of your face looking up at me exuding innocence and pure love is what got me through those weeks I had to be away from you and Tuscan. It nearly killed me to not be able to hold you, kiss you goodnight and hear your chatter and laughter. But, being reunited with you and all the love you poured out that you had saved up during our time apart made it all worthwhile.

You see being a Mommy is a lot of work. That is just the truth. I am choosing to be honest with you. To me, it's the best way to be. But it is a precious privilege. I see you playing "Mommy" a lot with your baby dolls. I know you would like to be a Mommy some day. If that is God's plan for you, I know you will do a wonderful job. You have a lot of love and affection to give to your lucky little babies.

I want to be a wonderful Mommy to you. I am not perfect. Like I've said to you before, just like you are learning to be a sweet and obedient little girl, I am learning to be a good Mommy. It's scary to realize that you are a little soul that will live forever, if you are guided in the right direction. I pray that I will be a safe example to follow and that you will also be inspired by all the other ladies that are a part of your life to be the best kind of girl and eventually woman you can possibly be.

I love you to Europe and back—driving, (your line!)

Your Mommy

LETTER TO WAYNE

You are most definitely not guilty. I hate that my mind made you into something you were not. But, it made my reality a very welcome, sweet thing to step back into.

Thank you for demonstrating that love is patient and love is kind. I have not been the easiest person to live with. I am sure, after all you witnessed, it's hard to trust that I am capable of all the things you expect of a wife and Mother. So, thank you for being willing to wait for me to regain ground and reassume responsibility. We have been through the fire and because of that, the gold in our marriage has been purified and the unnecessary fluff that we thought was important has disappeared.

I am amazed that you remained standing and upright during the horrendous month I "left" you. But, pillars are tested and appreciated for what they are when weight bears on them. You have proven your strength.

You are a terrific daddy. Our children adore you and for good reason.

Thank you for loving me and sticking by my side, for better or for worse,

Your Wife

MY PARTING SOAP BOX

I have a lot to learn about Motherhood. I will not pretend that I know anything more than the next mom. But, one thing I learned through my postpartum experience was that I need time and space away from my children.

Okay, I've said it.

This does not mean I am a bad mom.

This does not mean I am selfish.

This does not mean I resent them.

It means that I need to fill up my Mommy "tank" by stepping away and letting qualified, trusted people, be it a friend, family member, spouse, or hired nanny, take over my mom duties on a temporary and/or ongoing basis. It's good for me and it's good for my kids. Sometimes all that is needed is a few hours at a coffee shop, running errands solo or exercising. I need breaks. I need to just be "me" with no little beings dependent on me. Time away gives me the opportunity to miss them and to step back and realize how much I love them. Most importantly, it's great medicine for my mental health.

I have observed peers who refuse to trust another individual with their babies. I respect their choice, but am saddened when they let themselves get run down, lose their patience and resent that they don't have time to themselves.

No one loves your kids like you. True. And there are some people who are not to be trusted—your gut will tell you who they are and who to stay away from. But, look around. There are so many wonderful caregivers who have a lot of love, skill and wisdom to share with you and your kids.

Another excuse I have heard from Mothers is that they cannot afford help. Bologna! Exchange with another Mom. Bartering is brilliant!

Open yourself up to help. There can be a lot of joy and blessing when your child-raising journey is shared with others who have "been there and done it." I truly believe that it takes a village to raise and child!

Lastly, and most importantly, pray! We can't do this Motherhood thing on our own and in our own, often-unreliable strength. I have learned to pray for patience with my kids, my spouse and myself. I have begged for contentment in my current situation and to not wish away my kids' current stage of development. I pray for wisdom to guide tender souls. I pray to find joy in mundane housekeeping tasks. And, I have learned that God loves to give these things when asked. His gifts have increased my faith and have made me thankful in the deepest measure.

A HAPPY ANNIVERSARY

One year ago today I insanely ran down the street with my baby in my arms. One year ago I distrusted everyone who loved me most. One year ago I acted on a primal, yet delusional instinct to save my precious babies and run away from the evil in the world.

Here I sit in the now-famous recliner wrapping up this book. Home sweet home. Wayne is at work. Talia is having a swim day at preschool until three o'clock. Tuscan is jabbering himself to sleep in his crib. I feel whole, happy and partly healed. I don't know if someone is ever the same after a experiencing a bout of insanity. I would like to think I have changed, that I have a deeper understanding of what it looks and feels like to be in the depths of despair, alone and vulnerable.

I think of those fragile human vessels, each with a heart and a soul, confined to psych wards—cold, impersonal, sterile walls with maximum security. I pray that God would hear the groanings of their souls and give them rest from their demons. I pray that He would keep them safe from others and from themselves. I pray that they might be healed with the chemicals that can restore balance, that they find the rest they need to recover, and that they be filled courage and hope that they can be whole again.

The weather is partly sunny and a few clouds dot the sky. Much the way Motherhood is. A mix of joy and sorrow. Of fear and faith. Of worry and wonder. Of confidence and cries for help.

I've shed a few tears today. They come from a thankful, relieved heart. I am one fortunate Mommy to have survived a potentially devastating postpartum illness. The experience makes one realize how fragile our minds and our bodies really are. We were wonderfully and fearfully made.

59350075R00129

Made in the USA
Lexington, KY
02 January 2017